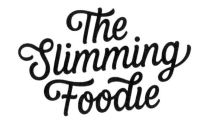

EASY MEALS
EVERY DAY

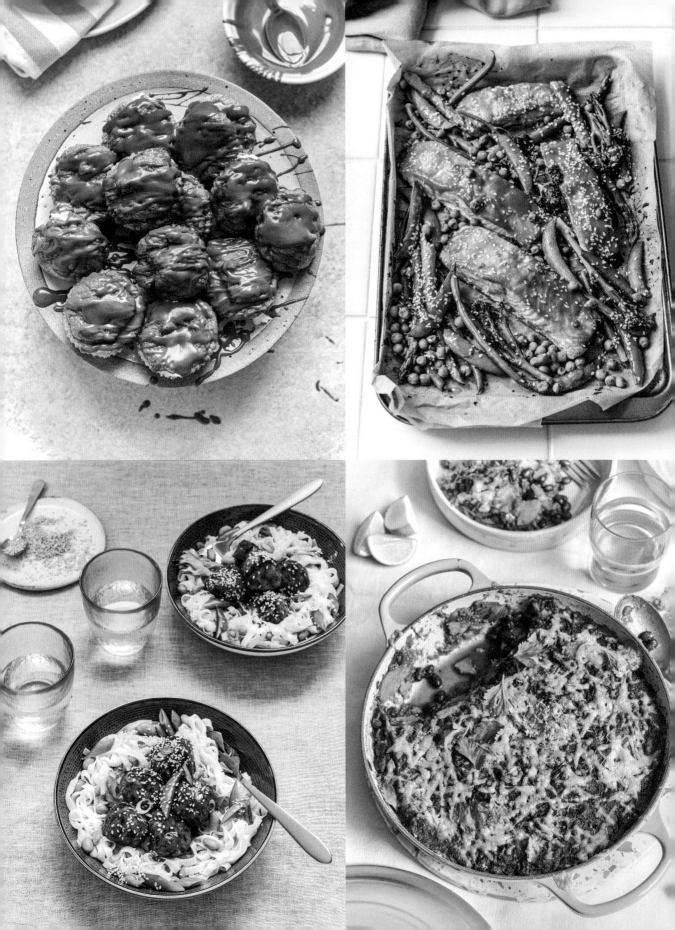

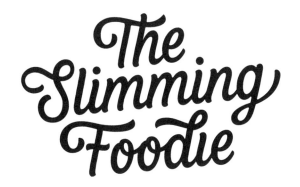

The Slimming Foodie

EASY MEALS EVERY DAY

Healthy dinners for the whole family

PIP PAYNE

hamlyn

hamlyn

First published in Great Britain in 2024 by Hamlyn,
an imprint of Octopus Publishing Group Ltd
Carmelite House, 50 Victoria Embankment
London EC4Y 0DZ
www.octopusbooks.co.uk

An Hachette UK Company
www.hachette.co.uk

Distributed in the US by Hachette Book Group
1290 Avenue of the Americas
4th and 5th Floors, New York, NY 10104

Distributed in Canada by Canadian Manda Group
664 Annette St., Toronto, Ontario, Canada M6S 2C8

ISBN 978 1 78325 565 8

A CIP catalogue record for this book is available from the
British Library.

Printed and bound in China
10 9 8 7 6 5 4 3 2 1

Editorial Director: Natalie Bradley
Senior Managing Editor: Sybella Stephens
Copy Editor: Lucy Bannell
Art Director: Yasia Williams
Design concept: www.gradedesign.com
Photographer: Chris Terry
Food Stylist: Henrietta Clancy
Props Stylist: Tamsin Weston
Production Controllers: Lucy Carter & Nic Jones

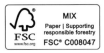

AUTHOR'S NOTES:

The information contained in this book is not intended to replace any
dietary advice from your own qualified nutritionist or dietician. Any
application of the ideas and information contained in this book is at
the reader's sole discretion and risk.

Both imperial and metric measurements have been given in all recipes.
Use one set of measurements only and not a mixture of both.

 Suitable for vegetarians

 Freezer friendly

CONTENTS

INTRODUCTION 6

1
Meat-Free Monday
12

2
Trays-Out Tuesday
34

3
Whip-It-Up Wednesday
58

4
Thrifty Thursday
84

5
Feasting Friday
112

6
Sumptuous Saturday
136

7
Staples Sunday
160

8
Something Sweet
184

9
Lucky Dip
206

MEAL PLANS 228

RECIPE LIST 232

INDEX 236

GLOSSARY 240

ACKNOWLEDGEMENTS 240

INTRODUCTION

One of the loveliest things about releasing a cookbook is seeing the food come to life in homes all around the world. Because my books all spring from the support of my amazing social media communities, I am lucky enough to see this phenomenon where photos, videos and stories are shared with me every single day, showing which of my recipes you have all been cooking.

It's exciting for me, when a book is first released, to find out which dishes most capture your imaginations. Within days, I can discover which are the most popular recipes, and this then helps me to learn the types of meals that I should focus on in future.

I am a home cook – I'm not trained as a chef – but I think this is an advantage in creating recipes for other home cooks. What a chef might consider simple or obvious isn't necessarily *either* of those things to someone who cooks at home. My focus has always been on making meals as easy as possible, cutting out unnecessary steps and getting maximum flavour with minimum fuss. And, of course, my particular priority is in thinking of ways that I can increase the nutrition content and cut out unnecessary fat and sugar. I also always want to make meals as budget-friendly as possible, while their ingredients should be easy to source in supermarkets for anyone who isn't able to regularly pop by an Italian deli. (Nothing against Italian delis, I absolutely love them, but my nearest one is an hour-and-a-half round trip!)

One thing I have noticed, after the release of each of my last three books, is how many people create weekly meal plans using only my recipes. I see books with day-of-the-week page dividers from Monday through to Sunday, each marking a different meal. I think it's absolutely wonderful that my dishes are able to provide inspiration for every day of the week, and that is what gave me the seed of the idea for this book. I have thought about the days of the week and what types of recipes might be useful for each specific day, and here's what I came up with:

Meat-Free Monday

Many people now observe meat-free Monday as a way of being more mindful of their meat consumption, so I've included lots of delicious vegetarian recipes in this chapter. You will also find plenty of vegetarian recipes scattered through other chapters too, as well as loads of notes suggesting swaps for the meat in my dishes or how to adjust recipes to make them vegetarian.

Trays-Out Tuesday

Who doesn't love a traybake? As the busy week ramps up, here are some easy, throw everything in, oven-baked recipes.

Whip-It-Up Wednesday

For most people, time is of the essence for weekday mealtimes, so here are some super-quick ideas to get a nutritious meal on the table in a flash, with plenty of family-favourite dishes.

Thrifty Thursday

This chapter focuses on budget-friendly meals, although as this is a subject uppermost in my mind, every other chapter has affordable options, too.

Feasting Friday

I have always loved to eat something special on a Friday night, so this chapter focuses on fakeaway options which will beat any takeaway!

Sumptuous Saturday

On a Saturday, many of us can take a little more of a leisurely pace with cooking, so here are a few ideas for some meals which might take a little extra time or effort for a really exceptional result, or which you might like to cook on a special occasion for friends or family.

Staples Sunday

I always like us to eat together as a family on a Sunday, so this chapter has some classic family favourites, as well as slow-cooker recipes. Many of these dishes will also leave you with some leftovers to help you out for meals during the following week.

Something Sweet

We can't forget the odd sweet treat or dessert. My philosophy is that, if you are going to have a treat, it should actually *be* a treat, not a pale imitation. So, though I try to cut down on fat and sugar as much as I can to make these recipes healthier, they still hit the spot as an occasional indulgence. I have also included some bakes that are great fun to cook along with kids and which you can enjoy eating with them, too.

Lucky Dip

Here are all the extra bits and bobs, from side dishes to spice mixes, to help you out on your daily food journey and make your cooking life easier.

I really hope that you find this book as easy and practical to use as I intended. And please continue to share with me what you have cooked at home!

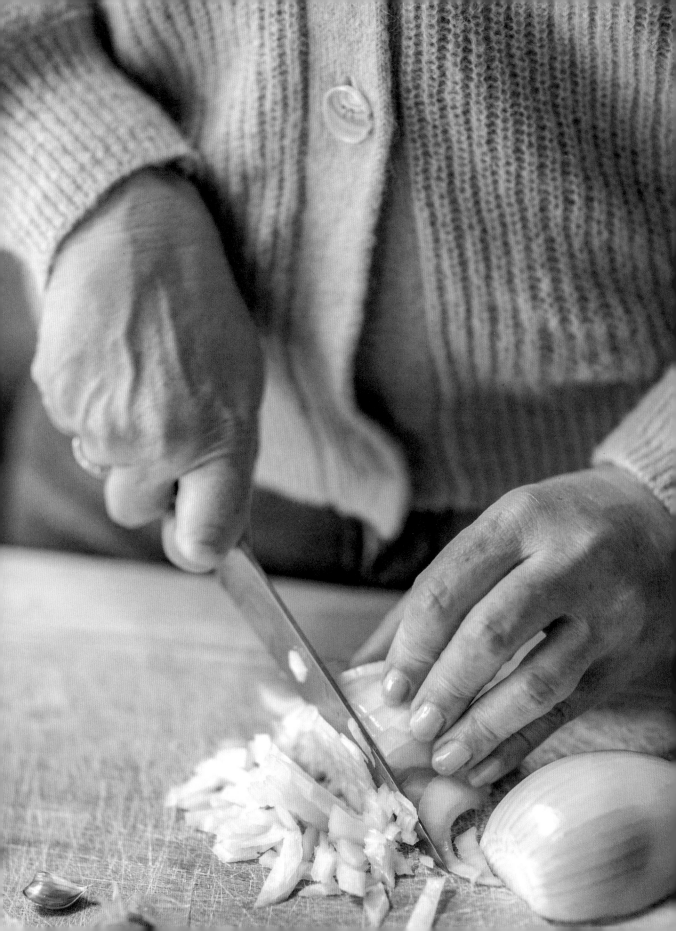

STORE CUPBOARD

The way to get good, fast flavour into food is by having a well-equipped store cupboard. As you begin to cook these recipes, your store cupboard will grow and you'll find there are many ingredients that are used regularly. If I have suggested buying a more specialist ingredient, I try to ensure that it is used in at least two meals in the book (and you may find it's used in my other *Slimming Foodie* books, too), so you can make the most of it and it isn't wasted. I'm not going to list every ingredient you might need here, as I think the best way for you to proceed is to mark the recipes you most want to cook and build up your store cupboard from there.

ESSENTIAL KIT

You don't need anything fancy or expensive to be able to make great meals at home, but there are a few essentials which just make life in the kitchen a lot more practical. Here are my suggestions:

EQUIPMENT

A good, sharp knife
You will use this every day, so if you can afford to, invest in a good one. *Keep it sharpened*: a blunt knife will both mean that food preparation takes so much longer and leave you more at risk of cutting yourself as you try to hack through things.

Measuring spoons
A lot of ingredients in these recipes use spoon measures to help you to get the quantities right.

Kitchen scales
To keep the calorie counts accurate, you'll need to stick to the weights given in the recipes.

Large mixing bowl

Microplane grater
A little bit more of a 'luxury' utensil, I use mine so often for zesting fruit and grating Parmesan cheese that it really is worth the investment.

Garlic press

Meat thermometer

Pots, pans and dishes

Sauté pan with a lid
Probably my most-used pan, because it's great for frying, but also has space for a whole curry if need be!

A *casserole dish with a lid*
I have an enamelled shallow casserole which, although heavy, I find useful for meals which involve both frying and oven-cooking.

Roasting tins
I have basic, stainless-steel roasting tins in three sizes, which pretty much cover everything. I also have a couple of nonstick baking sheets.

Ovenproof dishes
I have both round and rectangular stoneware dishes. These pretty much cover most meals, including frittatas, lasagne and oven-baked pasta and rice dishes.

Cake tins
Loaf tin (900g/2lb) I'm a big fan of loaf cakes, so if you want to bake from the sweet chapter, you'll need one of these.

Nonstick square cake tin (23cm/9 inch)

12-hole muffin tin

APPLIANCES

Mini chopper
Probably my most-used gadget, this will come in handy for many of the recipes in the book. No need for anything fancy, mine is very basic and it does the job perfectly well.

Food processor
I use mine to whizz up sauces and dips and for large amounts of grating, plus for blending jobs that my stick blender isn't quite strong enough to handle.

Stick blender
An essential for soups. Again, there's no need for anything high spec; I find that the most basic model will do.

Slow-cooker
I have a basic, 3.5-litre (3.7-quart) slow-cooker, which works well for a family of four.

GENERAL NOTES

Prep and cook times
This is literally the time it takes to chop, grate or mix. I'm not an expert chopper, so these timings are for an intermediate home cook.

Ovens and hobs vary hugely
I used a budget induction hob and fan oven to test each recipe in this book. I keep a thermometer in my oven to make sure I can give you an accurate reflection of the temperatures I'm cooking at. The failsafe check to ensure meat is cooked properly is to use a meat thermometer.

Fresh garlic and ginger
I generally use fresh garlic or ginger rather than tubes or pastes as I think the taste is better, plus there are no preservatives. If you are really in a rush, then there's no harm in using a ready-made paste. I also use the paste for my Slow-cooker Ginger Beer Ham (see page 171), as it gives better coverage in a glaze.

Salt
I often specify 'coarse ground salt', which just means I'm not using table salt, as a teaspoon of that will give a different level of salty taste. My preferred salt is Cornish sea salt flakes, partly because I'm from the West Country and I like that it's local to me, but also because it crumbles nicely when sprinkling over food.

Oil
I mainly use spray oil in my cooking, but I also use low-calorie cooking spray when I need better coverage, mainly for oven-cooking. In some recipes, I suggest a spoon measure of oil, because the recipe just requires that little bit extra for success.

Eggs
All eggs used are large, free-range eggs.

Light and reduced-fat ingredients
The recipes in this book are designed to be lower in fat and calories, but I know that many people who enjoy cooking from my books are not watching either of those. Please feel free to use a full-fat version of any light and reduced-fat ingredients, such as sausages, coconut milk and cream cheese. I love the fact that my recipes are enjoyed by all!

Pans and dishes used
If I think it matters, I will suggest a certain type of pan or dish. If you use something different, then cooking times may vary.

Food prep
The best way to cook a successful meal is to prep your ingredients in advance, as well as quickly reading through the full recipe before you start to make sure there aren't any surprises!

Calories
The calorie counts I provide are for a single portion and do not include serving suggestions or side dishes not in the ingredients list. If an ingredient is listed as 'optional', it isn't included in the calorie count. Calorie calculations can vary based on the precision of measurements, the brand of ingredients (for example, cans of light coconut milk can vary in calorie content), or the source of your nutritional data. The information provided here is intended as a guide.

Portion sizes
This is a very hard thing to generalize: a family with two toddlers is going to need a very different amount of food from a family with two teenagers! I base my portion sizes on recommended amounts, as well as on my experience of making the dish, and what I consider to be a satisfying portion. Of course, this is very subjective, and you may need to adjust these to work for you and your family. It's always worth cooking some extra vegetables on the side for filling-power if you think you may need them! I also realize that not every household is made up of four people, so you will find that many of the recipes are easy to scale up or down, and it's also great to be able to freeze leftover portions for another day.

Freezing
I make suggestions for freezer-friendly food based on what I would freeze, and what I know will defrost and reheat well. You may well be able to freeze other meals, but they may change consistency when reheated, which is why I have not marked them as freezer-friendly. When freezing meals, always allow the food to fully cool before placing it in the freezer. Transfer leftovers into airtight plastic containers or freezer bags, then label them with the contents and date. Make sure that food is thoroughly defrosted before reheating.

Symbols
Look out for these symbols at the top of each recipe:

  Suitable for vegetarians

  Freezer-friendly

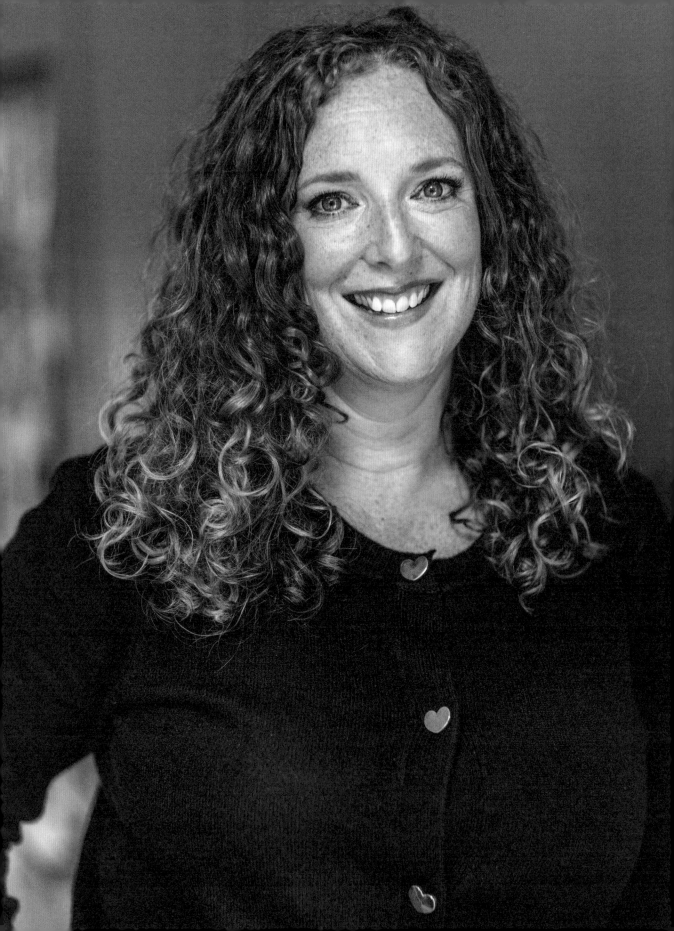

- ✔ SWEET POTATO AND MOZZARELLA 'SAUSAGE' ROLLS
- ✔ BALSAMIC ONION AND FETA FRITTATA
- ✔ BUTTERNUT SQUASH AND SPINACH LASAGNE WITH RICOTTA SAUCE
- ✔ OVEN-BAKED LEEK AND PEA RISOTTO
- ✔ GNOCCHI TOPPED VEGGIE COTTAGE PIE
- ✔ INDIAN 5-SPICE SWEET POTATO CURRY
- ✔ QUINOA, POMEGRANATE, WALNUT AND FETA SALAD
- ✔ BULGUR WHEAT, ROASTED MUSHROOM AND ROCKET SALAD
- ✔ CAULIFLOWER CHEESE AND JALAPEÑO SOUP
- ✔ LENTIL AND KALE SOUP

Meat-Free Monday

1

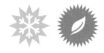

SWEET POTATO & MOZZARELLA 'SAUSAGE' ROLLS

MAKES 12
PREP TIME: 10 MINUTES
COOK TIME: 30 MINUTES

2 sweet potatoes (total weight about 500g / 1lb 2oz)

spray oil

2 onions, finely chopped

2 garlic cloves, crushed

1 teaspoon dried rosemary

1 teaspoon chilli flakes

100g (3½oz) mozzarella, grated

plain flour, to dust

2 filo pastry sheets

1 egg, lightly beaten

salt and pepper

Soft sweet potato and melted mozzarella with a crisp layer of filo pastry make these just as satisfying as a regular sausage roll. They make easy picnic food, and my youngest daughter loves them in her packed lunch.

You can eat these warm or cold and they will store in an airtight container for up to 4 days in the refrigerator (the pastry will not retain its crunch, but they will still be delicious). A great way to reheat them and crisp up the pastry again is to heat them in an air fryer for about 5 minutes.

1 Preheat the oven to 200°C/180°C fan (400°F), Gas Mark 6.

2 Prick the sweet potatoes a few times with a fork, place on a microwave-safe plate and microwave for 5 minutes. Pierce all the way through with a sharp knife: if they still feel a bit hard, microwave in 30-second bursts until they are tender all the way through.

3 Meanwhile, spray a frying pan with oil and place over a medium-low heat. Fry the onions for about 10 minutes, stirring often, then add the garlic and rosemary for the last minute of cooking.

4 Cut the sweet potatoes in half and scoop the flesh out into a bowl. Mash with a fork. Add the fried onions and chilli flakes, season with salt and pepper, then stir through the mozzarella.

5 Lightly dust a work surface with flour and lay down the 2 filo pastry sheets, one on top of the other. With a sharp knife, cut the filo pastry in half lengthways. Take half the sweet potato mixture and roll it into a sausage shape with your hands (you might have to do this in 2–3 steps). Lay each sausage along each filo pastry strip, lengthways.

6 Brush one long edge of each piece of filo with beaten egg, then fold the unbrushed long edge of the pastry over the sweet potato sausage and press down gently but firmly on the egg-washed side. You should have 2 very long sausage rolls. Cut each into 6 even pieces with a sharp knife.

7 Line a large baking tray with nonstick baking paper and carefully transfer the rolls to the tray (filo pastry can be prone to splitting). Brush each roll with the remaining beaten egg, then bake for 20 minutes, until the pastry is golden brown and crisp.

PER ROLL
CALORIES 99
FAT 2.3G
SAT FAT 1G
CARBS 15G
SUGARS 4G
FIBRE 1.7G
PROTEIN 3.9G
SALT 0.31G

> For a slightly more indulgent – and more robust – treat, swap the filo pastry for puff pastry.
> You can mix up the type of cheese you use: feta works well, or try Cheddar or red Leicester.
> If you fancy adding a bit of meat, fry some small bits of smoked bacon or chorizo and mix this in with the mashed sweet potato.

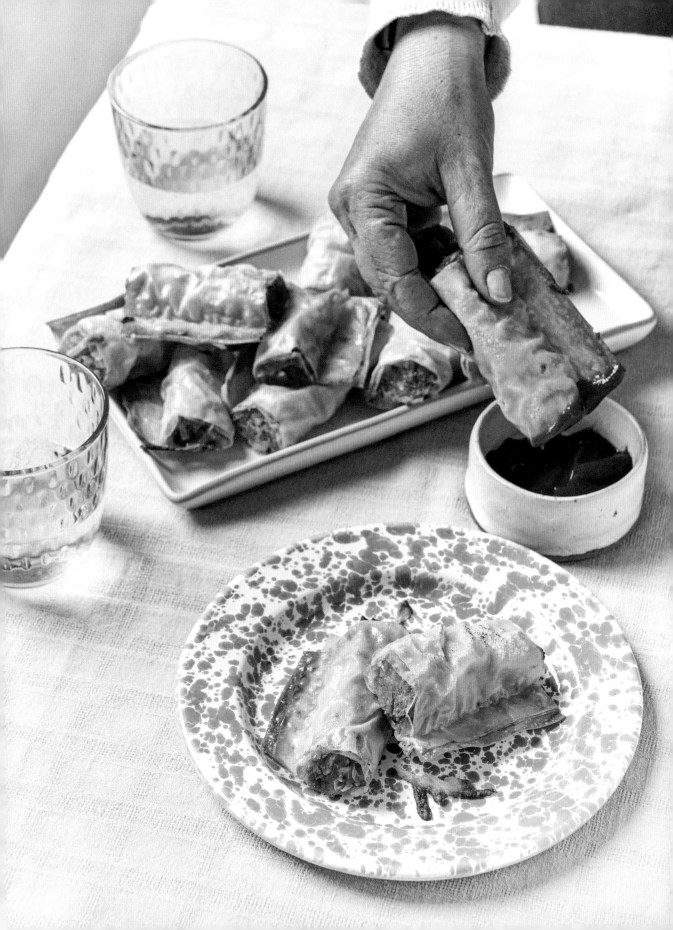

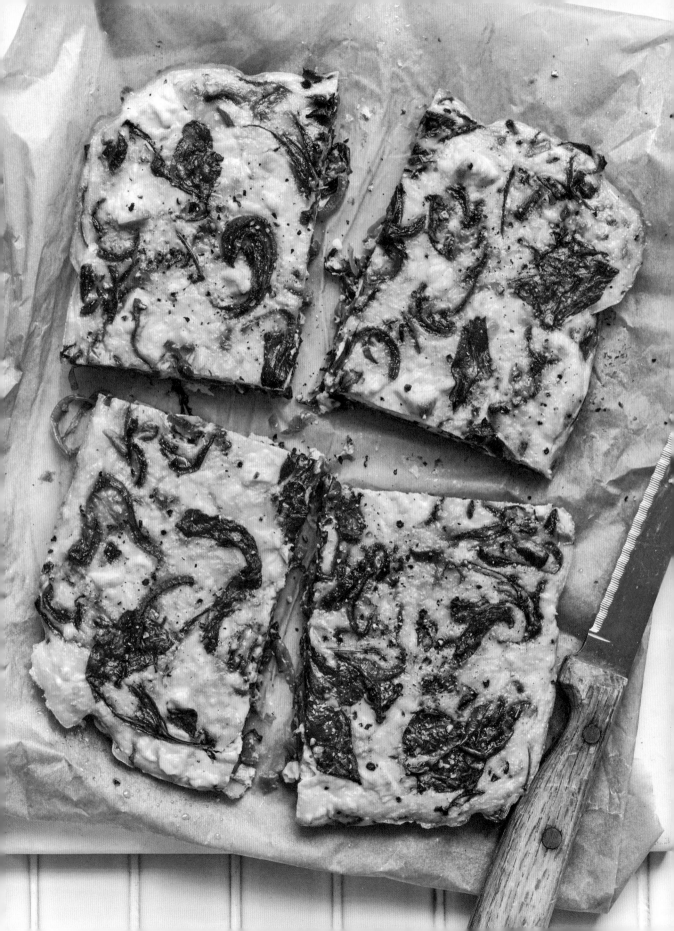

BALSAMIC ONION & FETA FRITTATA

SERVES 4
PREP TIME: 10 MINUTES
COOK TIME: 40 MINUTES

spray oil

3 red onions, halved and finely
   sliced into half moons

2 tablespoons balsamic vinegar

1 tablespoon honey

2 large handfuls of baby spinach
   leaves

½ teaspoon dried thyme

6 eggs

90g (3¼oz) feta cheese, crumbled

salt and pepper

Balsamic onions work so well in this simple dish. Frittatas are brilliant either for a filling main meal, or you can eat them cold for easy lunches or picnics.

1   Preheat the oven to 180°C/160°C fan (350°F), Gas Mark 4.

2   Spray a frying pan with oil and place over a low heat. Fry the onions gently for 12 minutes until they are soft, then stir in the balsamic vinegar and honey and cook for another minute. Stir in the spinach and thyme, then remove the pan from the heat.

3   In a bowl, lightly beat the eggs with salt and pepper, then add the crumbled feta.

4   Line a tin or baking dish with nonstick baking paper (I use a 20cm/8 inch square tin). Spoon in the fried onion mixture and spread evenly over the bottom, then pour in the egg mixture and tilt the tin to spread the egg around evenly.

5   Bake on the middle shelf of the oven for 25 minutes.

6   Lift out of the tin, cut into 4 and serve.

PER SERVING
CALORIES 233
FAT 13G
SAT FAT 5.3G
CARBS 14G
SUGARS 10G
FIBRE 1.1G
PROTEIN 16G
SALT 1.2G

Note

There are a huge variety of balsamic vinegars available, with an equally huge range of prices! Investing in a good-quality balsamic is worth it for the extra flavour you get. At the more expensive end of the scale, balsamic vinegar is thick and sweet, so if yours is thin and sour, it's not the best sort. In the UK, I love the Belazu brand, which is a great mid-priced balsamic vinegar.

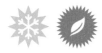

BUTTERNUT SQUASH & SPINACH LASAGNE

SERVES 4
PREP TIME: 20 MINUTES
COOK TIME: 55 MINUTES

1 large butternut squash (around
  1kg / 2lb 4oz), peeled and cut into
  1cm (½ inch) cubes

250g (9oz) cherry tomatoes, halved

4 garlic cloves, crushed

2 tablespoons tomato purée

1 teaspoon coarse ground salt

½ teaspoon freshly ground black
  pepper

1 teaspoon finely chopped sage
  leaves

150g (5½oz) baby spinach leaves,
  roughly chopped

250g (9oz) ricotta cheese

180ml (6fl oz) semi-skimmed milk

45g (1½oz) vegetarian Parmesan-
  style cheese, finely grated

180g (6oz) dried lasagne sheets
  (around 10 sheets)

150ml (¼ pint) hot vegetable stock

A simple but tasty vegetarian lasagne with a creamy and mild ricotta sauce. This is an ideal dish to make up in advance, then just bake when you want it, which makes it great for dinner parties and family get-togethers. Serve this up with a simple green salad if you would like something on the side.

1   Preheat the oven to 220°C/200°C fan (425°F), Gas Mark 7.

2   Put the squash in a large mixing bowl with the tomatoes, garlic, tomato purée, salt and pepper and sage and mix them all together. Add the spinach and mix it into the other ingredients.

3   Make up the ricotta sauce in another bowl by mixing together the ricotta, milk and 25g (1oz) – or roughly half – the Parmesan.

4   In a baking dish or tray (I use a rectangular dish measuring 28 x 23cm/ 11 x 9 inches), layer in half the butternut squash mix. Roughly snap half the lasagne sheets into pieces about 5cm (2 inches) across and arrange it over the squash. Breaking up the pasta helps the sheets to evenly cover the surface area and makes the lasagne easier to portion up once it's cooked.

5   Now spoon half the ricotta sauce over the broken-up lasagne, using the back of the spoon to gently spread it around to cover as much of the pasta as possible.

6   Add the rest of the butternut squash mix and spread it into an even layer. Pour the hot vegetable stock over the top and then cover with the remaining lasagne sheets, snapping them in pieces as before. Spoon over the rest of the ricotta sauce, spread it around to cover the pasta, then finish by evenly sprinkling the remaining Parmesan over the top.

7   Bake the lasagne on the middle shelf of the oven for 10 minutes, to allow the cheese on top to melt and brown a little so it won't stick to foil. Remove the dish from the oven, cover tightly with foil (be careful here not to burn your hands, use oven gloves or a tea towel), then return the lasagne to the oven and bake for 45 minutes.

PER SERVING
CALORIES 436
FAT 10G
SAT FAT 5.9G
CARBS 61G
SUGARS 20G
FIBRE 8.2G
PROTEIN 21G
SALT 1.7G

> You can use frozen butternut squash cubes for this if you prefer, but they may not be cut as small, so you will need to allow a longer cooking time for them to defrost and cook through: add an extra 15 minutes to the time that you cook the lasagne under the foil. You may just want to test a squash cube when you take the lasagne out of the oven, too, to make sure it is fully cooked.

> If you like the idea of adding meat to this dish, a sprinkling of thinly sliced pancetta added to the middle layer gives great, complementary flavour.

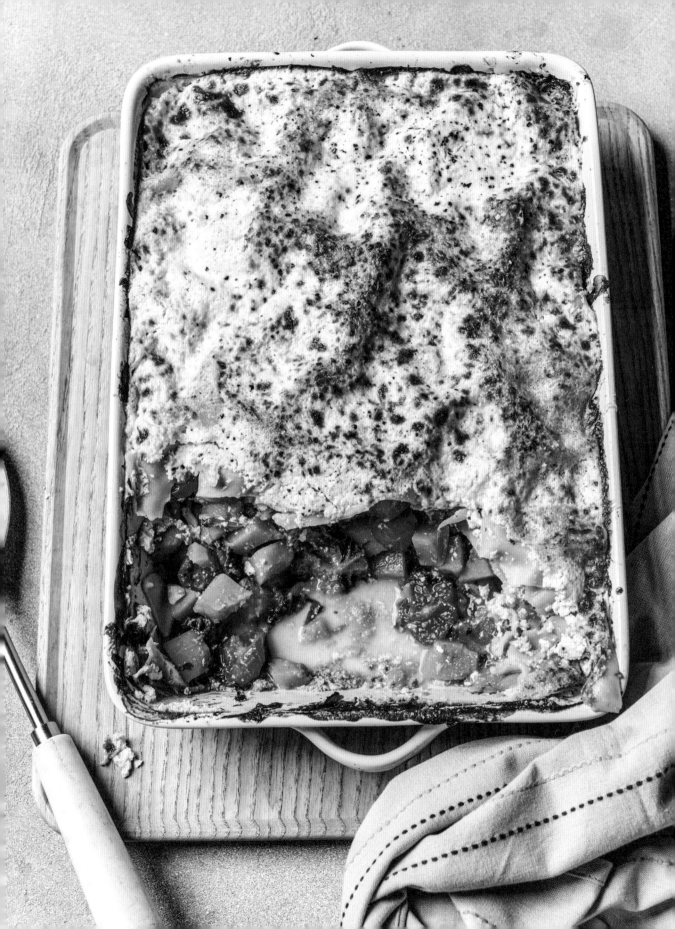

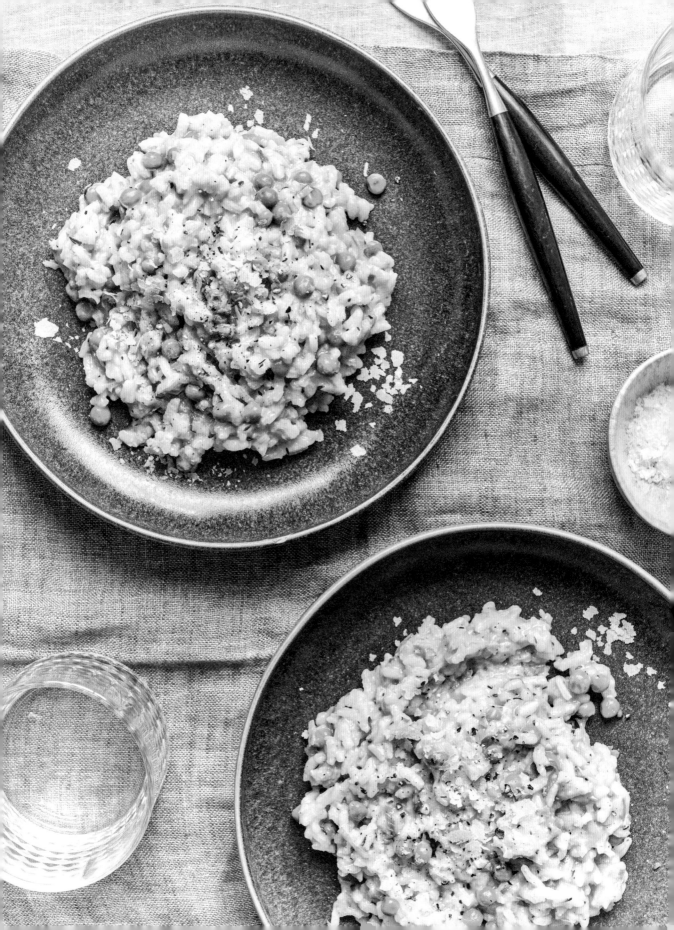

OVEN-BAKED LEEK & PEA RISOTTO

SERVES 4
PREP TIME: 10 MINUTES
COOK TIME: 30 MINUTES

spray oil

2 leeks, trimmed, cleaned and thinly sliced

2 garlic cloves, crushed

1 teaspoon dried thyme

250g (9oz) arborio rice

800ml (1 pint 8fl oz) hot vegetable stock

1½ tablespoons nutritional yeast (reserve some for a garnish)

juice of ½ lemon

200g (7oz) frozen petits pois

salt and pepper

Take the hassle out of making risotto by baking it in the oven. The simple flavours here create a warming and satisfying meal.

1 Preheat the oven to 200°C/180°C fan (400°F), Gas Mark 6.

2 Spray a flameproof and ovenproof casserole, which has a tightly fitting lid, with oil, then fry the leeks over a medium heat for 5 minutes. Add the garlic and thyme and cook for another minute. Add the rice and cook with the vegetables for about 2 minutes.

3 Pour in 600ml (1 pint) of the vegetable stock and season with salt and pepper. Bring up to a simmer, stir, put the lid on and place on the middle shelf of the oven for 10 minutes.

4 Remove from the oven, stir, add the remaining vegetable stock, nutritional yeast, lemon juice and frozen petits pois, stir well, place the lid back on and cook in the oven for a further 10 minutes.

5 Try a bit of rice to check it's fully cooked through and doesn't have a grainy texture. If it's still got a bit of a bite, pop it back in the oven for another 5 minutes. Serve with the reserved nutritional yeast sprinkled on top.

Note

PER SERVING	
CALORIES	405
FAT	3.5G
SAT FAT	0.9G
CARBS	69G
SUGARS	12G
FIBRE	13G
PROTEIN	17G
SALT	0.37G

If you haven't used nutritional yeast before, it's a great ingredient for adding savoury flavour to vegetarian and vegan dishes. If you buy a tub to use for this recipe, make sure it doesn't just languish in the cupboard! Here are some other ways to use it:

> Sprinkled over pasta, salad or casserole as an extra seasoning, or stirred through soups and casseroles.

> As a cheesy flavour in vegan sauces.

> As an alternative thickener to cornflour for soups, stews and sauces.

> Mixed into seasonings and spice mixes for an extra layer of flavour.

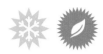

GNOCCHI-TOPPED VEGGIE COTTAGE PIE

SERVES 4
PREP TIME: 15 MINUTES
COOK TIME: 1 HOUR
10 MINUTES

spray oil

2 onions, chopped

2 celery stalks, finely chopped

2 carrots, finely chopped

2 garlic cloves, crushed

1 large sweet potato (350g / 12oz), peeled and chopped

125g (4½oz) dried red lentils

4 tablespoons tomato purée

1 tablespoon miso paste

1 teaspoon sweet paprika

1 litre (1¾ pints) vegetable stock

3 large handfuls of baby spinach leaves

500g (1lb 2oz) fresh gnocchi

60g (2¼oz) Cheddar cheese, grated

salt and pepper

finely chopped flat leaf parsley, to garnish

One of the things that sometimes puts me off making cottage pie is the step of cooking mashed potato, so I decided to experiment with a gnocchi topping… and I loved it! The gnocchi turns soft inside with a bit of crunch on top, and it is such an easy way to top a pie without any labour.

1   Spray a large flameproof and ovenproof pan with oil, place over a medium heat and fry the onions, celery and carrots for 10 minutes. Stir in the garlic, sweet potato, lentils, tomato purée, miso paste and paprika and cook for 1 minute.

2   Pour in the vegetable stock and simmer gently for 35 minutes. When there are 10 minutes remaining, preheat the oven to 210°C/190°C fan (410°F), Gas Mark 6½.

3   Stir in the spinach leaves and season with salt and pepper.

4   Arrange the gnocchi on top, sprinkle the cheese evenly over and bake for 25 minutes. Scatter with chopped parsley to garnish.

PER SERVING
CALORIES 513
FAT 8G
SAT FAT 4.3G
CARBS 82G
SUGARS 18G
FIBRE 11G
PROTEIN 22G
SALT 2.6G

Note

Frozen potato waffles can also make a quick and easy cottage pie topping. Simply swap out the gnocchi for the waffles, although it might be best to transfer the filling to a large rectangular baking dish, to create more surface area for the waffles.

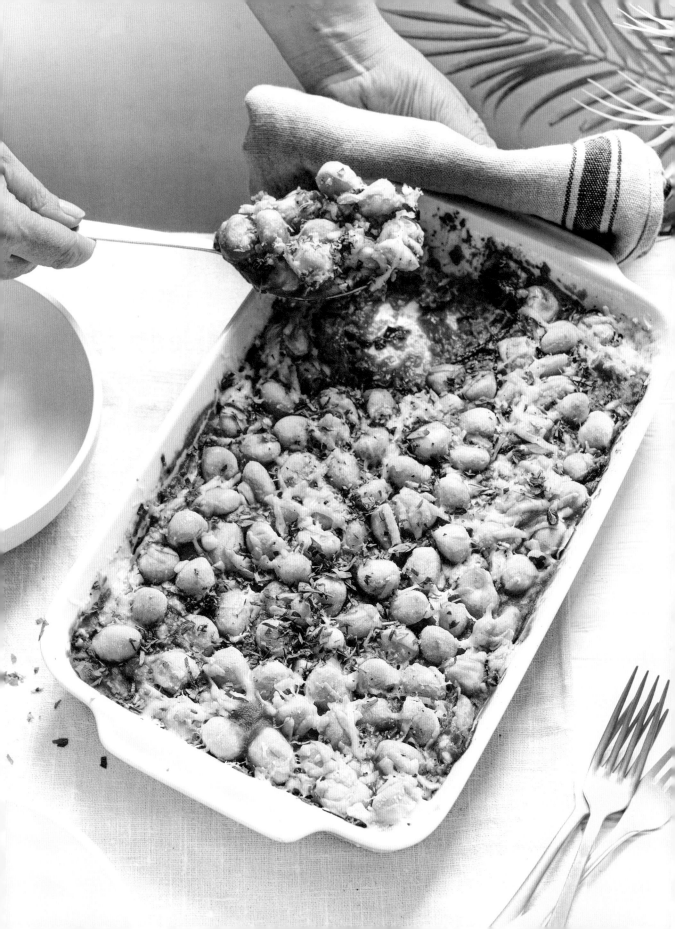

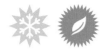

INDIAN 5-SPICE SWEET POTATO CURRY

SERVES 6
PREP TIME: 10 MINUTES
COOK TIME: 35 MINUTES

1 tablespoon vegetable oil

2 onions, finely chopped

2 tablespoons Indian 5-spice Blend (see page 225)

3 garlic cloves, crushed

1 litre (1¾ pints) hot vegetable stock

2–3 medium-large sweet potatoes (total weight 750g / 1lb 10oz), peeled and chopped

150g (5½oz) dried red lentils

400ml (14fl oz) can of reduced-fat coconut milk

1 teaspoon coarse ground salt

300g (10½oz) frozen spinach

A satisfying, creamy curry made with toasted spices for real depth of flavour. This is a brilliant curry which is quick to put together (especially if you have your Indian 5-spice Blend ready, see page 225). This serves 6 as it is great for feeding a group, but it's also ideal to reheat for easy lunches, so it is always worth making a bigger batch.

1   Heat the oil in a large, flameproof casserole, add the onion and cook, stirring, for 5 minutes.

2   Add the Indian 5-spice and the garlic, then cook for another minute.

3   Pour in the stock, then add the sweet potatoes and lentils. Stir in the coconut milk and salt, then leave to simmer for 25 minutes, stirring every now and again.

4   Add the frozen spinach, leave to simmer for another 5 minutes, stir well to incorporate the spinach into the sauce and serve.

PER SERVING
CALORIES 361
FAT 11.3G
SAT FAT 5.1G
CARBS 46.3G
SUGARS 12G
FIBRE 9.4G
PROTEIN 13.9G
SALT 1.1G

Note

This isn't a hot curry, so if you want to add some heat, stir in some finely chopped fresh chilli, or chilli flakes, when you add the spice and garlic in step 2. You can really add any extra veggies you fancy: fry some chopped red pepper with the onions, add butternut squash with the sweet potatoes, or add quicker-cooking vegetables such as cauliflower and broccoli florets, green beans or peas for the last 10 minutes of cooking time. If you'd like to add meat, you can fry some chopped skinless chicken or lamb with the onions, or for a seafood twist, add cooked, peeled prawns for the last 10 minutes of cooking.

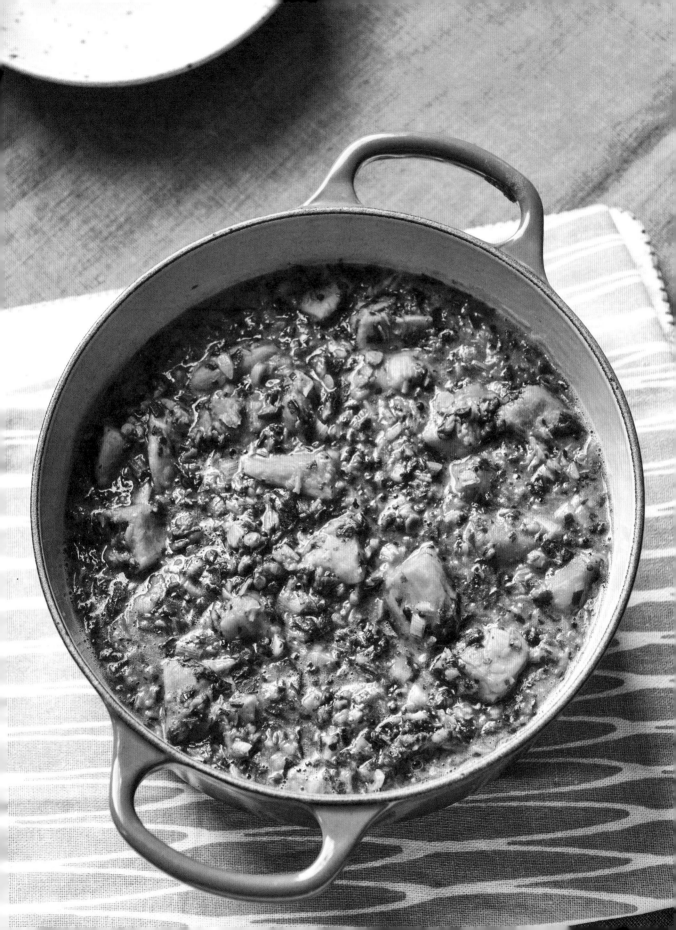

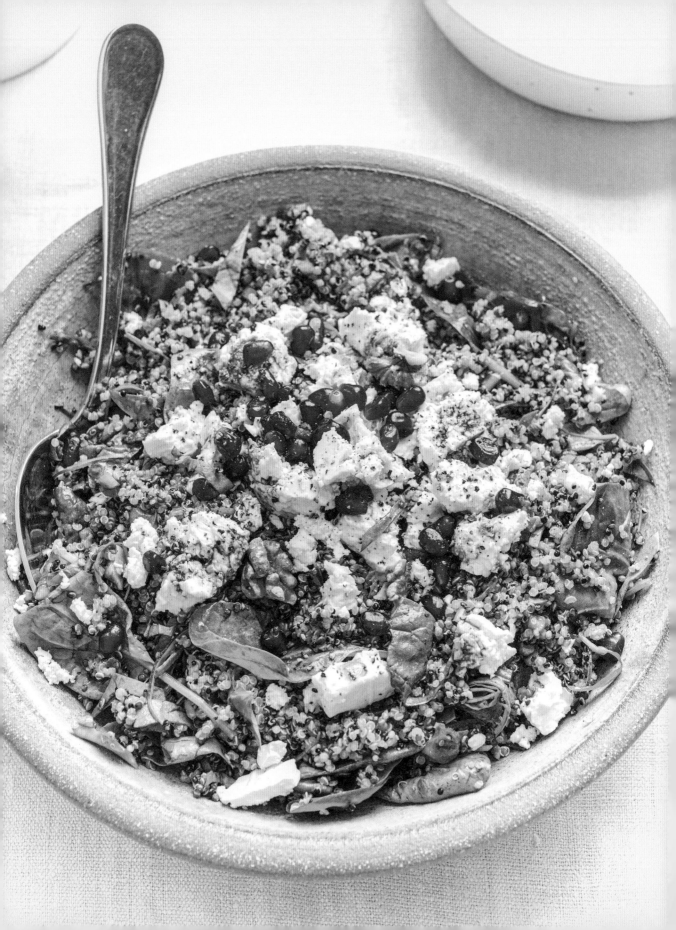

QUINOA, POMEGRANATE, WALNUT & FETA SALAD

SERVES 4
PREP TIME: 10 MINUTES
COOK TIME: 15 MINUTES

200g (7oz) red, white or mixed colour quinoa

50g (1¾oz) walnuts, roughly chopped

¼ red onion, very finely sliced

150g (5½oz) baby spinach leaves, roughly chopped

50g (1¾oz) pomegranate seeds

90g (3¼oz) feta cheese, crumbled

FOR THE BALSAMIC DRESSING

2 tablespoons balsamic vinegar

1 tablespoon olive oil

1 tablespoon honey

2 teaspoons Dijon mustard

1 garlic clove, crushed

½ tsp coarse ground salt

½ tsp freshly ground black pepper

A delicious and filling dish which is quick to throw together and packed full of flavour and texture.

1. Cook the quinoa according to the packet instructions (usually 10–15 minutes), then drain and leave to cool while you prepare the rest of the ingredients.

2. In a frying pan, dry-fry the walnut pieces for about 4 minutes to toast them.

3. Transfer the quinoa to a large bowl, add the red onion and walnuts, then toss to mix.

4. Make up the balsamic dressing by shaking all the ingredients together in a jar.

5. Add the spinach to the quinoa mixture along with most of the pomegranate seeds and half the feta. Drizzle over the balsamic dressing and toss again until the dressing is fully combined.

6. Top with the rest of the crumbled feta and the remaining pomegranate seeds and serve immediately.

PER SERVING
CALORIES 345
FAT 16G
SAT FAT 4.3G
CARBS 33G
SUGARS 3.8G
FIBRE 5.2G
PROTEIN 14G
SALT 1.4G

Note

If you are preparing this in advance, don't add the balsamic dressing until you are ready to serve, or it will wilt the spinach. You could also add more vegetables to the salad: try grated beetroot or carrot, finely chopped parsley leaves, rocket or chopped cucumber.

BULGUR WHEAT, ROASTED MUSHROOM & ROCKET SALAD

SERVES 4
PREP TIME: 10 MINUTES
COOK TIME: 20 MINUTES

250g (9oz) raw bulgur wheat

6 spring onions, finely sliced

40g (1½oz) rocket, roughly chopped

1 red chilli, deseeded and finely chopped

large handful of parsley leaves, finely chopped

juice of ½ lemon

salt and pepper

FOR THE ROASTED MUSHROOMS

250g (9oz) chestnut mushrooms, sliced

250g (9oz) large flat mushrooms, halved, then sliced

1 tablespoon olive oil

3 rosemary sprigs

¼ teaspoon coarse ground salt

½ teaspoon freshly ground black pepper

2 garlic cloves, crushed

This salad is filling and satisfying, with garlic-roasted mushrooms giving it real depth of flavour. A bowl of this is a meal in itself, although it also makes a great side dish to other salads, meats or cheeses: try serving it with some griddled halloumi, or mini mozzarella balls. This is delicious served warm or cold.

1   Preheat the oven to 220°C/200°C fan (425°F), Gas Mark 7.

2   Start by preparing the roasted mushrooms. Mix up the sliced mushrooms in a large bowl with the olive oil, rosemary sprigs and salt and pepper, then tip into a baking tray and spread out evenly. Place on the middle shelf of the oven to roast for 20 minutes, giving them a good stir twice during the cooking time.

3   Meanwhile, cook the bulgur wheat according to the packet instructions and prepare the rest of the vegetables.

4   When the mushrooms have 5 minutes remaining, stir through the crushed garlic and pop back into the oven for the final bit of cooking time.

5   Once the bulgur wheat is cooked, drain and set aside to cool.

6   Remove the mushrooms from the oven and discard the rosemary sprigs.

7   Place the bulgur wheat in a large bowl, fluff it through with a fork, then stir through the roasted mushrooms, spring onions, rocket, chilli, parsley and lemon juice. Season with salt and pepper.

PER SERVING
CALORIES 293
FAT 4.8G
SAT FAT 0.7G
CARBS 49G
SUGARS 1.8G
FIBRE 5.9G
PROTEIN 11G
SALT 0.58G

Note

Salads like this are brilliant for using up bits and pieces: you could mix up the grains by using quinoa or couscous, or add extra chopped-up vegetables and herbs such as cherry tomatoes, cucumber, baby spinach, courgette, green beans, mint or coriander. Roast some small chorizo cubes or diced bacon along with the mushrooms for a meaty twist, or add leftover cooked and shredded chicken or pork.

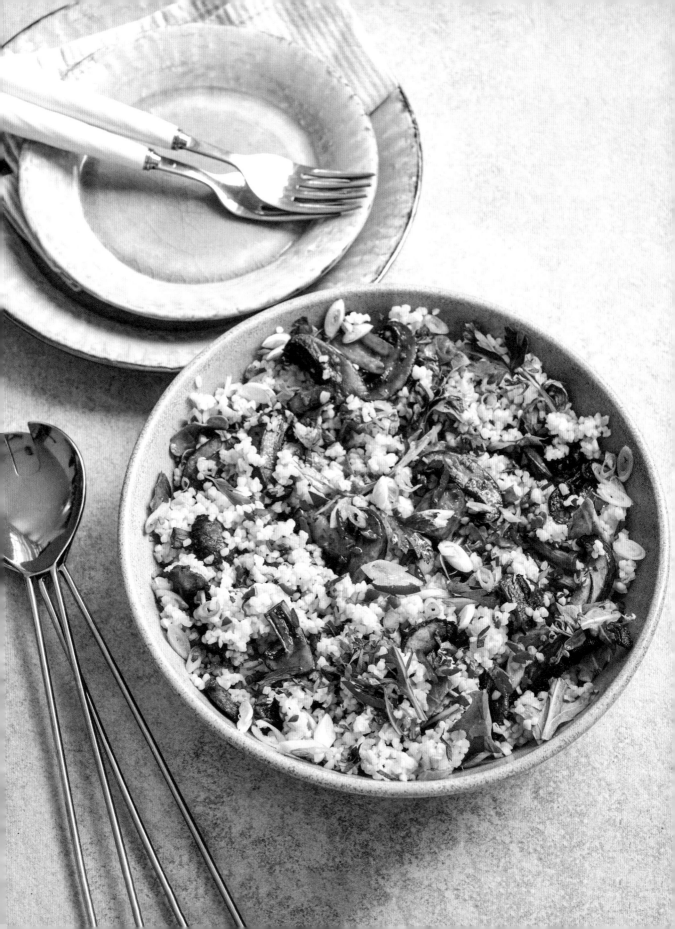

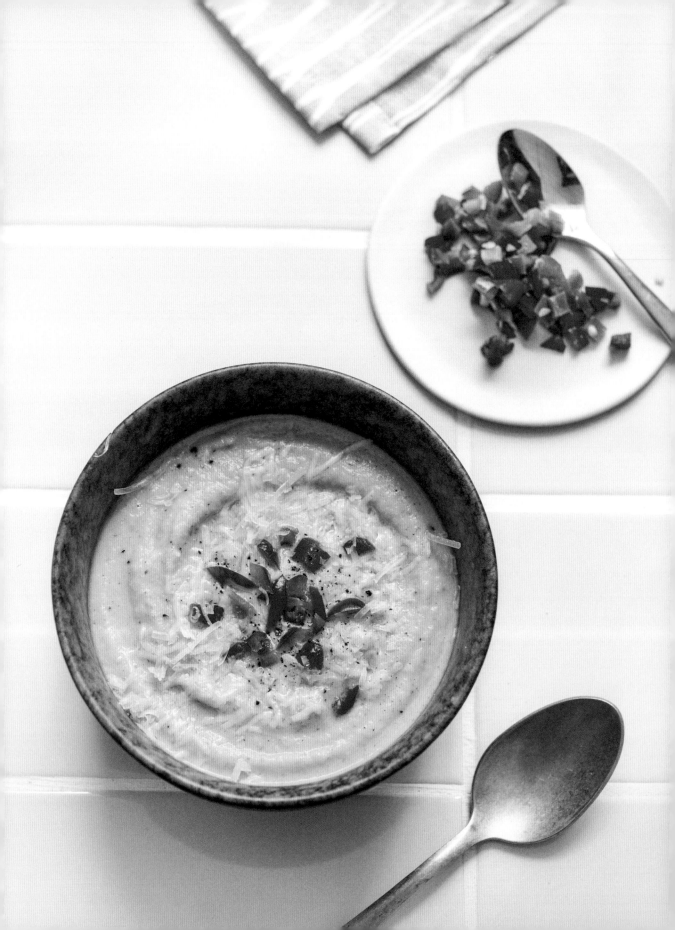

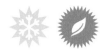

CAULIFLOWER CHEESE & JALAPEÑO SOUP

SERVES 2
PREP TIME: 5 MINUTES
COOK TIME: 30 MINUTES

spray oil

1 medium-large cauliflower, broken into florets

1 onion, chopped

2 garlic cloves, crushed

1 tablespoon roughly chopped pickled jalapeños, plus extra to serve

500ml (18fl oz) hot vegetable stock

60g (2¼oz) mature Cheddar cheese, grated

¼ teaspoon coarse ground salt

¼ teaspoon freshly ground black pepper

A creamy, silky soup which is comforting and filling, with a subtle warming kick from the jalapeño. You can experiment with different cheeses such as Gruyère, Stilton or Roquefort, but if using a stronger cheese, start with a small amount and build the flavour to your taste, and omit the jalapeños.

1   Spray a sauté pan with oil and place over a medium-high heat. Stir-fry the cauliflower for 5 minutes, until it just starts to get slightly toasted on the edges.

2   Add the onion and fry for another 5 minutes, stirring occasionally, until it has softened. Add the crushed garlic and jalapeños and fry for 1 minute.

3   Pour in the hot stock, bring to the boil, then reduce the heat to a simmer and allow to simmer for 15 minutes.

4   Transfer to a large bowl or large jug and use a stick blender to blend it into a smooth and creamy soup.

5   Add the cheese and salt and pepper, stir to melt the cheese into the soup, then serve scattered with extra jalapeños if liked.

PER SERVING
CALORIES 308
FAT 13G
SAT FAT 7.3G
CARBS 29G
SUGARS 15G
FIBRE 8.5G
PROTEIN 17G
SALT 1.7G

> In the UK, cauliflower is in season from June to October. It becomes a lot more expensive outside that time, so this is a great vegetable to eat seasonally.
> You can easily scale up this soup to serve more people. If you want to put some effort into presentation, you can scatter it with finely chopped parsley leaves, spring onions or chives, or a few toasted cauliflower florets.

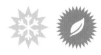

LENTIL & KALE SOUP

SERVES 4
PREP TIME: 10 MINUTES
COOK TIME: 35 MINUTES

spray oil

1 onion, chopped

2 celery stalks, sliced

3 garlic cloves, finely sliced

2 large carrots, chopped

1 teaspoon curry powder

400g (14oz) can of chopped
   tomatoes

1 litre (1¾ pints) hot vegetable
   stock

2 tablespoons tomato purée

2 teaspoons sweet paprika

1 teaspoon dried basil

1 teaspoon dried thyme

2 large handfuls of kale, coarse
   stems removed

400g (14oz) can of green lentils,
   drained and rinsed

juice of ½ lemon

salt and pepper

TO SERVE

chilli sauce, such as sriracha
   (optional)

crusty bread

chopped parsley

The perfect soup if you are feeling under par, this is full of goodness, warming and filling. I first made it to use up leftover kale, but it's now a regular in our household and there's always a couple of portions in the freezer.

1   Spray a large pot with oil, place over a medium-high heat and fry the onion, celery, garlic and carrots for 5 minutes. Stir in the curry powder and cook for 1 minute, then add the tomatoes.

2   Pour in the vegetable stock and add the tomato purée, paprika, basil and thyme. Stir, then simmer for 15 minutes.

3   Add the kale to the pot, simmer for 2 more minutes, then use a stick blender to blend into a smooth soup.

4   Add the lentils and simmer for 10 more minutes. Season with salt and pepper, then stir through the lemon juice and serve with a drizzle of chilli sauce over the top and some chopped parsley, if you like, with crusty bread on the side.

PER SERVING
CALORIES 190
FAT 3.1G
SAT FAT 0.7G
CARBS 25G
SUGARS 15G
FIBRE 10G
PROTEIN 8.9G
SALT 0.61G

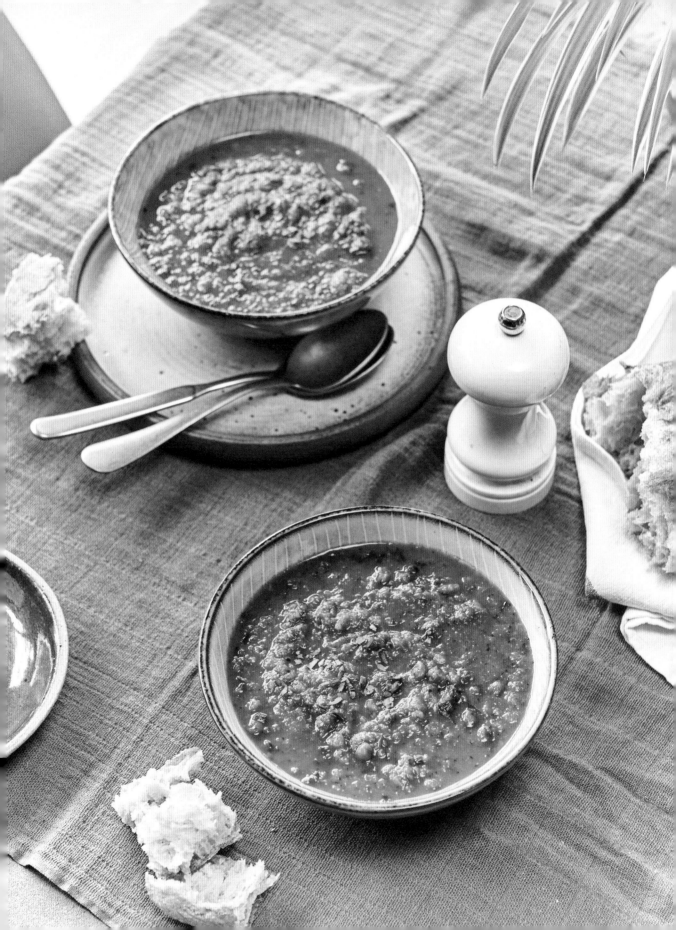

- ✓ BLACK BEAN AND CORN-LOADED QUESADILLAS
- ✓ ROASTED CARROT AND HARISSA SOUP
- ✓ SWEET POTATO AND BLACK BEAN LAYER
- ✓ KOREAN-STYLE SWEET CHILLI CHICKEN
- ✓ MISO-MAPLE GLAZED SALMON
- ✓ MEDITERRANEAN-STYLE FISH WITH GREMOLATA
- ✓ TERIYAKI CHICKEN TRAYBAKE
- ✓ INDIAN-SPICED CHICKEN AND VEG TRAYBAKE
- ✓ JALAPEÑO POPPER STUFFED COURGETTES
- ✓ BACON, LEEK, POTATO AND PEA BAKE
- ✓ LEMON AND GARLIC PORK WITH SWEET POTATO AND ONION WEDGES

2

Trays-Out Tuesday

BLACK BEAN & CORN-LOADED QUESADILLAS

SERVES 4
PREP TIME: 10 MINUTES
COOK TIME: 15 MINUTES

400g (14oz) can of black beans (in water), drained and rinsed

150g (5½oz) frozen sweetcorn

½ red onion, finely sliced

1 garlic clove, crushed

1 teaspoon smoked paprika

1 teaspoon dried oregano

finely grated zest of 1 lime

½ teaspoon ground cumin

2 tablespoons tomato purée

1 tablespoon finely chopped pickled jalapeños

120g (4½oz) Cheddar cheese, grated

4 plain tortilla wraps, or wholemeal/seeded wraps if you prefer

coriander leaves, to garnish

I was so pleased to discover this method of making a batch of quesadillas, because – although they make a quick, filling, nutritious and low-cost meal – making 4 in a row in a pan is way too time-consuming for me! Baking them like this allows you to make as many as you need to, all at once, and still gives you the perfect crisp outside and melty filling. On their own these make a great lunch or lighter meal, or add a salad, homemade coleslaw or chips on the side for a more filling option.

1   Preheat the oven to 220°C/200°C fan (425°F), Gas Mark 7.

2   Put all the ingredients – except the tortilla wraps – in a large mixing bowl and mix together thoroughly.

3   Place a tortilla on a large baking tray and cover half of it with one-quarter of the filling. Fold the other half of the tortilla over to form a semi-circle and cover the filling. Press down gently but firmly. You want the top half to stick down once everything starts to melt, but you don't want to squash all the filling out on to the tray.

4   Move the tortilla to the corner of the tray to make space for the rest and repeat with the other 3 tortillas (if your tray isn't big enough, then just do this over 2 baking trays).

5   Place on the middle shelf of the oven and bake for 7 minutes. The top should be mottled golden brown and crisp and the filling should be melty.

6   Remove the tray from the oven and, using a spatula, carefully flip over each quesadilla. If any filling falls out, just scoop it back in and use the spatula to gently press down on the top of the flipped quesadilla.

7   Place back in the oven and bake for another 5–7 minutes, until the top is also golden brown and crisp. Use a sharp knife to cut each quesadilla into half, then serve scattered with coriander leaves.

PER SERVING
CALORIES 406
FAT 15G
SAT FAT 8.1G
CARBS 43G
SUGARS 4.1G
FIBRE 9.1G
PROTEIN 19G
SALT 1.7G

Note

These quesadillas are loaded up, so are probably easier to eat with cutlery rather than with hands. If you want to make them easier to eat with hands, then just add a smaller amount of filling to each. This will also mean you can make more, or freeze some of the filling for another day.

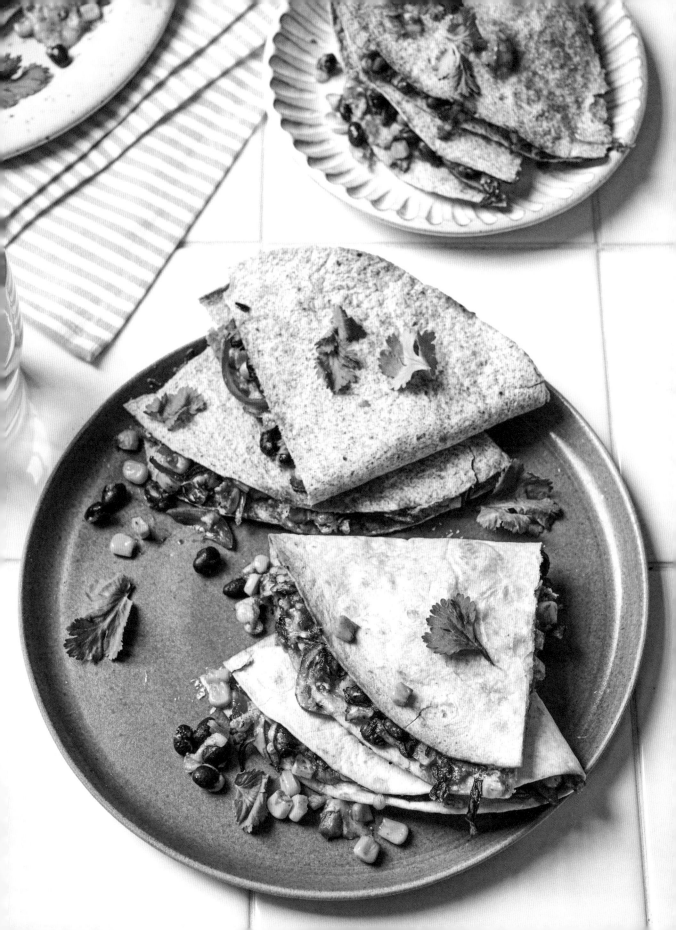

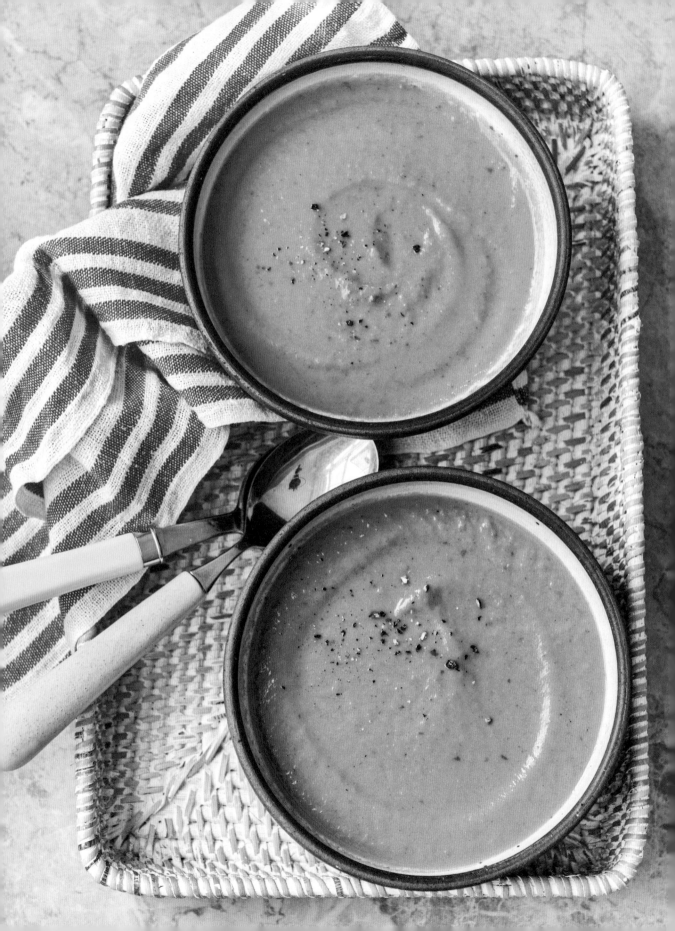

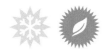

ROASTED CARROT & HARISSA SOUP

SERVES 4
PREP TIME: 10 MINUTES
COOK TIME: 40 MINUTES

900g (2lb) carrots, sliced

1½ teaspoons smoked paprika

spray oil, or low-calorie cooking
   spray

2 onions, chopped

2 garlic cloves, chopped

½ teaspoon ground cumin

¼ teaspoon cayenne pepper

400g (14oz) can of light coconut
   milk

700ml (1¼ pints) hot vegetable
   stock

2 tablespoons harissa paste

juice of ½ lemon

salt and pepper

**Roasting carrots adds such lovely depth of flavour to the vegetables
that it is really worth making that little bit of extra effort.**

1   Preheat the oven to 220°C/200°C fan (425°F), Gas Mark 7.

2   Place the carrots in a large roasting tin, sprinkle over ½ teaspoon of the
    paprika, spray with oil or low-calorie cooking spray, then mix well. Roast
    for 30 minutes, giving them a good shuffle around with a spatula halfway
    through cooking.

3   Meanwhile, spray a large pan with oil or low-calorie cooking spray and
    place over a medium-high heat. Fry the onions for 8 minutes, then add
    the garlic and stir-fry for another 1 minute. Add the cumin, cayenne and
    remaining 1 teaspoon paprika, stir well, then turn off the heat until the
    carrots are ready.

4   When the carrots have finished roasting, add them to the onion pan
    along with the coconut milk, vegetable stock and harissa paste.
    Simmer for 10 minutes.

5   Use a stick blender to blend into a smooth soup, add the lemon juice,
    season with salt and pepper and serve.

PER SERVING
CALORIES 239
FAT 10G
SAT FAT 6.9G
CARBS 27G
SUGARS 23G
FIBRE 12G
PROTEIN 3.9G
SALT 0.6G

Note

For any recipes that only use half a lemon, keep hold of the other half, cut it into quarters and
pop it into a freezer-safe sealed bag. Keep in the freezer for any time that you need a squeeze of
lemon juice. If you freeze it straight away, it saves it sitting around and going mouldy while you
forget about it!

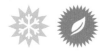

SWEET POTATO & BLACK BEAN LAYER

SERVES 4
PREP TIME: 15 MINUTES
COOK TIME: 1 HOUR
10 MINUTES

spray oil

2 red onions, chopped

3 garlic cloves, crushed

500g (1lb 2oz) tomato passata

4 tablespoons tomato purée

2 teaspoons dried oregano,
   plus more to serve

2 teaspoons smoked paprika

1 teaspoon ground cumin

1 teaspoon coarse ground salt

½ teaspoon freshly ground
   black pepper

2 medium sweet potatoes, peeled
   and thinly sliced (total weight
   about 600g / 1lb 5oz)

2 x 400g (14oz) cans of black
   beans, in water, drained
   and rinsed

1 lime, zested, then quartered

120g (4¼oz) Cheddar cheese,
   grated

coriander leaves, to garnish

A hearty vegetarian dish of fudgy sweet potatoes layered with black beans and a rich tomato sauce, with a subtly smoky, Mexican-inspired flavour.

1   Preheat the oven to 200°C/180°C fan (400°F), Gas Mark 6.

2   Spray a frying pan or sauté pan with oil, place over a medium-low heat and fry the onions for 8 minutes until soft. Add the garlic and stir through the onion for about 30 seconds. Add the passata, tomato purée, oregano, smoked paprika, cumin, salt and pepper. Stir well and bring to a simmer.

3   In a roasting dish (mine measured 30 x 20cm / 12 x 8 inches), spread out half the tomato sauce to cover the base. Add half the sweet potato slices, then half the black beans.

4   Sprinkle the lime zest over the black beans, then layer on the rest of the sweet potato, the remaining black beans and finally spoon over the second half of the tomato sauce, spreading it out to cover the whole dish.

5   Cover tightly with foil, then bake for 50 minutes.

6   Remove from the oven, sprinkle the cheese over the top, scatter on a few pinches of oregano, then bake uncovered for a final 10 minutes until the cheese is golden and bubbling. Serve scattered with a few coriander leaves.

PER SERVING
CALORIES 502
FAT 13G
SAT FAT 6.9G
CARBS 61G
SUGARS 27G
FIBRE 18G
PROTEIN 24G
SALT 2.7G

 Note

>   You can customize this to your tastes with favourite vegetables: add an extra layer of aubergine (cook it first to make sure it's soft, not chewy, see page 106), courgette or mushroom slices, or throw in some pickled jalapeños to ramp up the spice and flavour.

>   If you want to add some meat, fry some bacon, chorizo or sausage with the onions to include in the tomato sauce.

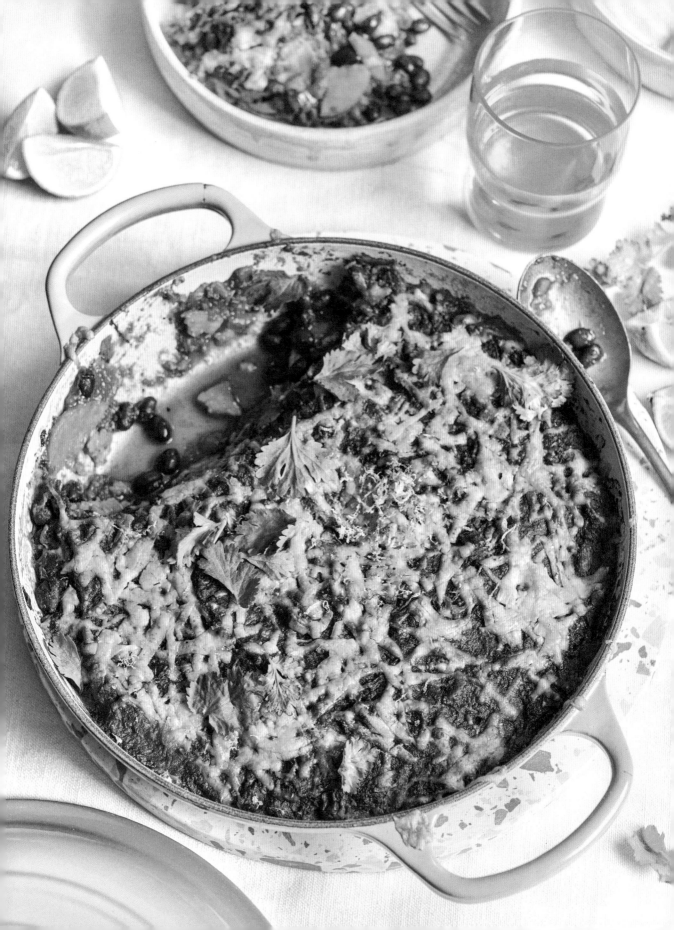

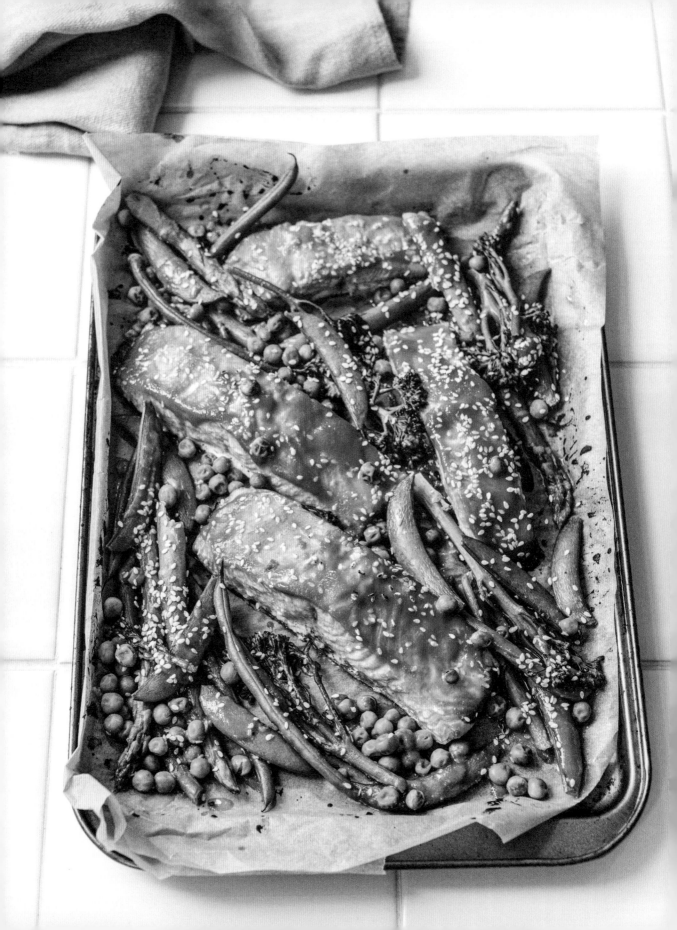

MISO-MAPLE GLAZED SALMON

SERVES 4
PREP TIME: 5 MINUTES
COOK TIME: 15 MINUTES

2 tablespoons white miso paste

1 tablespoon maple syrup

1 tablespoon mirin

1 tablespoon light soy sauce

½ teaspoon toasted sesame oil

4 salmon fillets

300g (10½oz) sugar snap peas

200g (7oz) frozen petits pois

1 teaspoon sesame seeds
   (black or white)

salt and pepper

Salmon fillets make a fabulous quick traybake and, in this recipe, a sweet-and-savoury glaze adds fantastic flavour... but only takes minutes to put together. I have used asparagus, green beans, sugar snap peas, broccoli and peas here, but you can substitute any quick-cooking vegetable, such as green beans, Tenderstem broccoli, asparagus, pak choi or mushrooms. For a more filling option, serve with a portion of Zakkoku Rice (see page 212).

1   Preheat the oven to 210°C/190°C fan (410°F), Gas Mark 6½.

2   Mix the miso, maple syrup, mirin, soy sauce and sesame oil together in a small bowl.

3   Place the salmon fillets together on one side of a large baking tray, and the sugar snaps and petits pois on the other side. Use a teaspoon to drizzle and spread the sauce over the salmon, then drizzle any remaining sauce over the vegetables. Season everything with salt and pepper and scatter the sesame seeds over the fish.

4   Place the tray in the oven and bake for 12–15 minutes (see note below), then serve

PER SERVING
CALORIES 397
FAT 22G
SAT FAT 3.9G
CARBS 14G
SUGARS 11G
FIBRE 4.6G
PROTEIN 33G
SALT 1.9G

Note

Salmon fillets can vary greatly in thickness and this will affect their cooking time. Thinner fillets are likely to take around 12 minutes, but allow 15 minutes for thicker-cut pieces. If you want to present the salmon with more of a golden-brown colour, set aside the vegetables in a warm bowl so they don't overcook, then pop the fish under a hot grill for a couple of minutes just before serving.

KOREAN-STYLE SWEET CHILLI CHICKEN

SERVES 4
PREP TIME: 10 MINUTES
COOK TIME: 30 MINUTES

4 skinless chicken breasts (total weight 600g / 1lb 5oz)

2 red, yellow or orange peppers, deseeded and chopped

100g (3½oz) sugar snap peas

150g (5½oz) cherry tomatoes, halved

2 red onions, each cut into 8 wedges

FOR THE SAUCE

2 tablespoons gochujang paste

2 tablespoons dark soy sauce

2 tablespoons tomato purée

1 tablespoon honey

1 tablespoon rice vinegar

2 garlic cloves, crushed

5 tablespoons water

TO SERVE

200g (7oz) mixed leaf salad, or crispy salad

½ cucumber, sliced

The sauce here is a real flavour explosion and a delicious way to turn a trayful of chicken and veg into something special. I serve this with a mixed salad.

1   Preheat the oven to 200°C/180°C fan (400°F), Gas Mark 6.

2   Spread the chicken, peppers, sugar snap peas, tomatoes and onions over the bottom of a baking tray.

3   Mix together all the sauce ingredients in a small bowl, then drizzle it all over the chicken and vegetables.

4   Place on the middle shelf of the oven and cook for 30 minutes.

5   Check that the chicken is cooked all the way through to the middle. Serve alongside the salad leaves and cucumber slices.

PER SERVING
CALORIES 290
FAT 2.8G
SAT FAT 0.6G
CARBS 22G
SUGARS 17G
FIBRE 4.7G
PROTEIN 41G
SALT 1.7G

Note

Gochujang is a Korean chilli paste which is thick, sticky and pungent. It is such a brilliant, flavoursome ingredient to have on hand, but I have found a real discrepancy in the taste of gochujang from different shops. Some supermarket own-brand gochujang is more like a sauce than a paste and does not pack half the flavour of an authentic version. Look out for a tub rather than a jar, and if you can make it to an Asian supermarket to find it, then all the better. You can also buy authentic brands online and in some supermarkets.

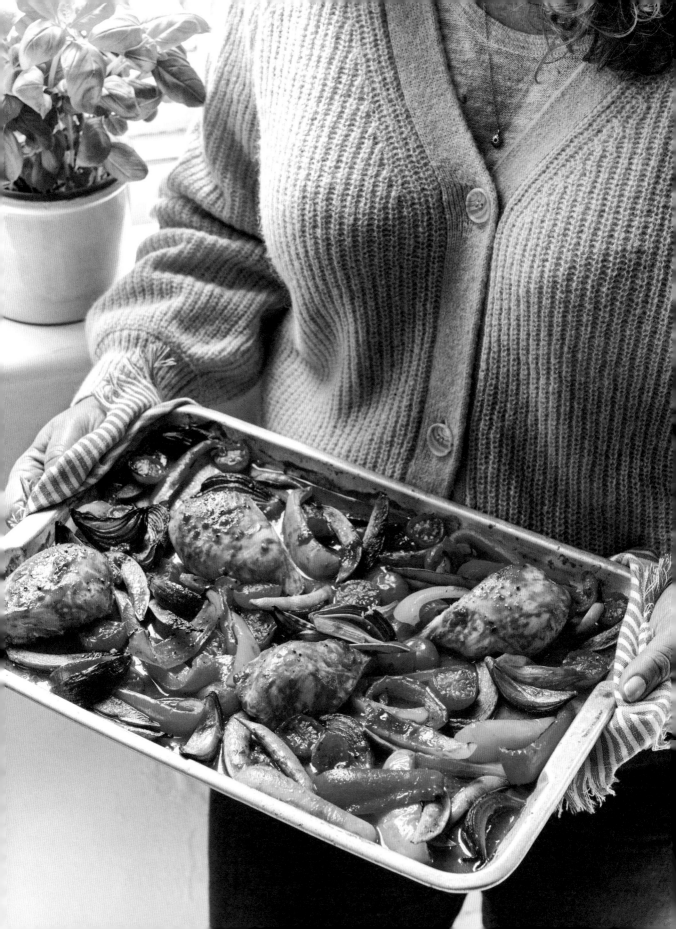

MEDITERRANEAN-STYLE FISH WITH GREMOLATA

SERVES 4
PREP TIME: 10 MINUTES
COOK TIME: 25 MINUTES

3 peppers (red, orange or yellow), deseeded and chopped

2 large courgettes, cut into half-moon slices about 5mm (¼ inch) wide

200g (7oz) cherry tomatoes

1 tablespoon olive oil

1 tablespoon balsamic vinegar

4 frozen white fish fillets

1 tablespoon dried mixed herbs

spray oil, or low-calorie cooking spray

200g (7oz) Tenderstem broccoli

salt and pepper

FOR THE GREMOLATA

30g (1oz) parsley leaves and stalks, very finely chopped

2 garlic cloves, crushed or finely grated

finely grated zest and juice of 1 lemon

The wonderfully healthy food of the Mediterranean inspired this dish, with its roasted vegetables and fish topped with fresh and zingy gremolata, an incredibly flavoursome mix of parsley, lemon and garlic.

1   Preheat the oven to 220°C/200°C fan (425°F), Gas Mark 7.

2   Put the peppers in a large baking tray with the courgettes and cherry tomatoes, then drizzle over the olive oil and balsamic vinegar and toss to coat the vegetables. Place the frozen fish among the vegetables, then scatter the mixed herbs over everything, season with salt and pepper and spray a little oil, or low-calorie cooking spray, over the top of each fish fillet.

3   Pop the baking tray on to the middle shelf of the oven and set a timer for 15 minutes.

4   Meanwhile, prepare the gremolata by combining all the ingredients in a bowl, adding a pinch of salt and mixing very thoroughly. Make sure that the parsley is as finely chopped as you can get it.

5   After 15 minutes, remove the baking tray from the oven, scatter over the broccoli and spritz a little spray oil, or low-calorie cooking spray, over the broccoli. Place back in the oven for another 10 minutes.

6   Divide between 4 plates and spoon the gremolata directly on to the cooked fish.

Note

PER SERVING
CALORIES 237
FAT 5.7G
SAT FAT 1G
CARBS 11G
SUGARS 10G
FIBRE 7.6G
PROTEIN 30G
SALT 0.53G

You can use any firm white fish of your choice here; most supermarkets sell packs of fish fillets which are great value and have been frozen while still lovely and fresh. Try the recipe with coley, cod, haddock, pollock or hake. The cooking time here is for thick frozen fish fillets. Depending on what fish you choose (and if you decide to use fresh rather than frozen) the time needed may vary, but you will find guidance on the fish packaging, or you can ask your fishmonger for a recommended cooking time. If you need to reduce the cooking time for the fish, then start the veg off first, so they can have the whole 25 minutes in the oven, then add the fish when a suitable cooking time remains.

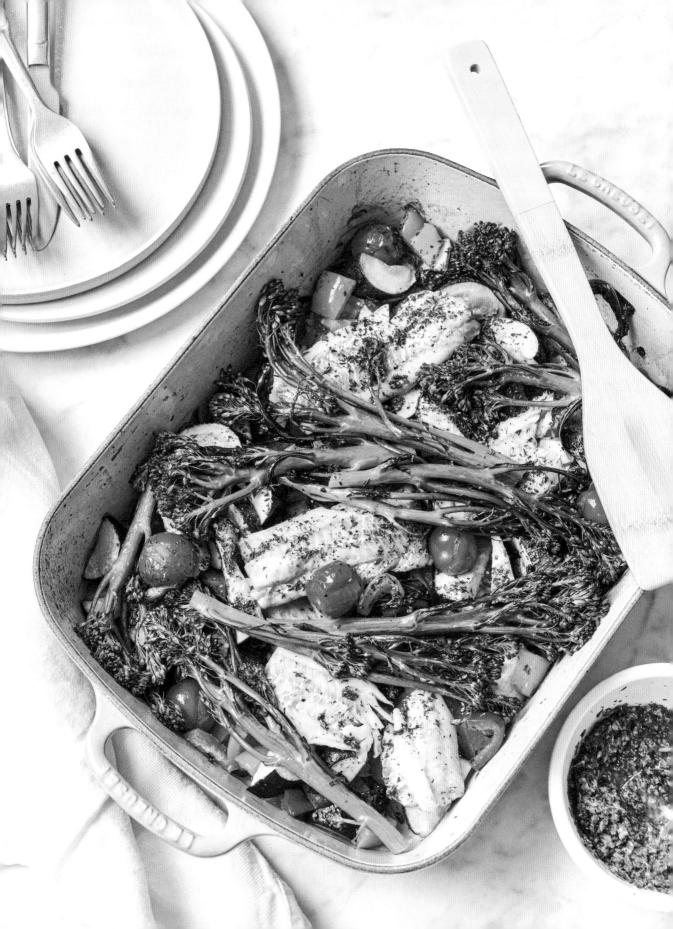

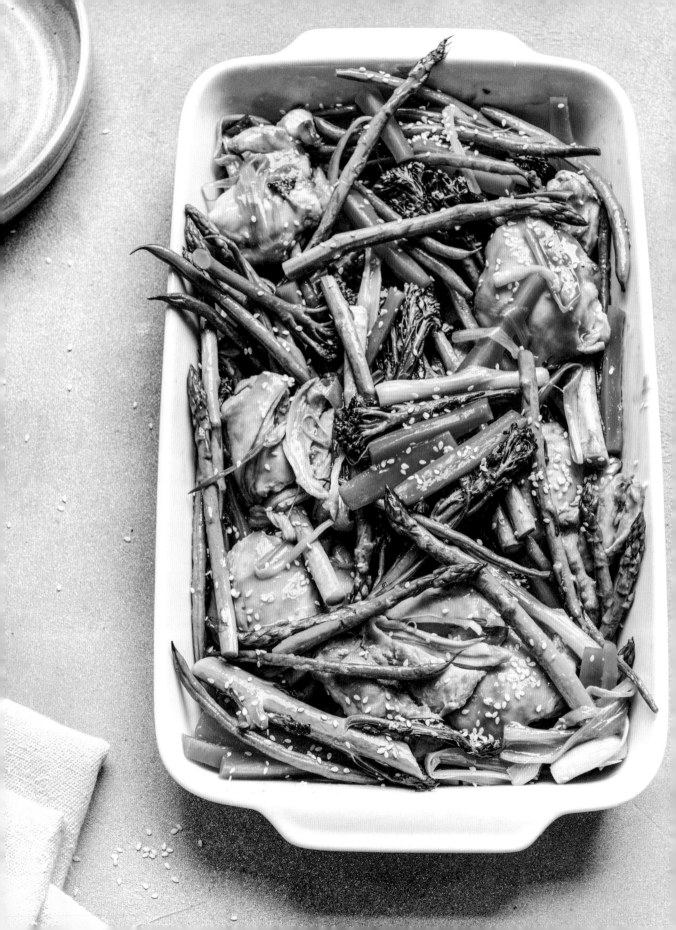

TERIYAKI CHICKEN TRAYBAKE

SERVES 4
PREP TIME: 10 MINUTES
COOK TIME: 35 MINUTES

2 carrots, sliced

8 spring onions, sliced

8 skinless chicken thigh fillets

6 tablespoons teriyaki sauce

150ml (¼ pint) water

150g (5½oz) asparagus spears, trimmed

100g (3½oz) fine green beans, topped and tailed

200g (7oz) Tenderstem broccoli

spray oil

salt

This simple recipe is a favourite in our house. You can use homemade Teriyaki Sauce (see page 227), or ready-made teriyaki sauce for ultra convenience. If you want to add a side dish, the Zakkoku Rice (see page 212) is perfect with this.

1   Preheat the oven to 200°C/180°C fan (400°F), Gas Mark 6.

2   Put the carrots and spring onions into a large baking tray and lay the chicken thigh fillets on top.

3   Mix the teriyaki sauce with the measured water, pour over the chicken and bake for 25 minutes.

4   Remove from the oven, add the asparagus, green beans and broccoli, spray with oil, sprinkle over a couple of pinches of salt, cover the tray tightly with foil and bake for another 10 minutes, by which time the vegetables should be tender.

5   Divide evenly between 4 plates.

PER SERVING
CALORIES 300
FAT 3.3G
SAT FAT 0.8G
CARBS 9.6G
SUGARS 8.3G
FIBRE 5.5G
PROTEIN 54G
SALT 3.2G

Note

For a vegetarian version, replace the chicken thigh fillets with large chunks of aubergine.

INDIAN-SPICED CHICKEN & VEG TRAYBAKE

SERVES 4
PREP TIME: 15 MINUTES
COOK TIME: 20 MINUTES

1 tablespoon olive oil

2 garlic cloves, crushed

1 tablespoon ground turmeric

1 teaspoon cumin seeds

1 teaspoon nigella seeds

finely grated zest and juice of
1 lemon

1 teaspoon coarse ground salt

¼ teaspoon freshly ground
black pepper

4 skinless chicken thigh fillets,
chopped small

1 red pepper, chopped

1 red onion, cut into wedges

1 cauliflower, cut into florets

400g (14oz) can of chickpeas,
drained

100g (3½oz) fat-free Greek yogurt

A simple but filling bake with chickpeas and cauliflower, served drizzled with a zesty lemon-yogurt dressing.

1   Preheat the oven to 200°C/180°C fan (400°F), Gas Mark 6.

2   In a small bowl, mix the oil, garlic, turmeric, cumin and nigella seeds, lemon juice and salt and pepper.

3   Spread the chicken, pepper, onion, cauliflower and chickpeas out in a baking tray, then drizzle the turmeric sauce all over. Mix the vegetables and chicken around so they are all coated in the sauce.

4   Bake for 20 minutes, giving everything a stir halfway through.

5   Meanwhile, mix the lemon zest and a pinch of salt into the yogurt. Use a teaspoon to drizzle the zesty yogurt over the top of the traybake before serving.

PER SERVING
CALORIES 345
FAT 7.3G
SAT FAT 1.2G
CARBS 27G
SUGARS 9.4G
FIBRE 7.3G
PROTEIN 41G
SALT 1.5G

Note

You can prepare this meal in advance by mixing the turmeric sauce, vegetables and chickpeas in a large lidded tub. You can then simply add the chicken, mix, tip it out into a baking tray and bake it when you need it, mixing up the zesty yogurt as it bakes.

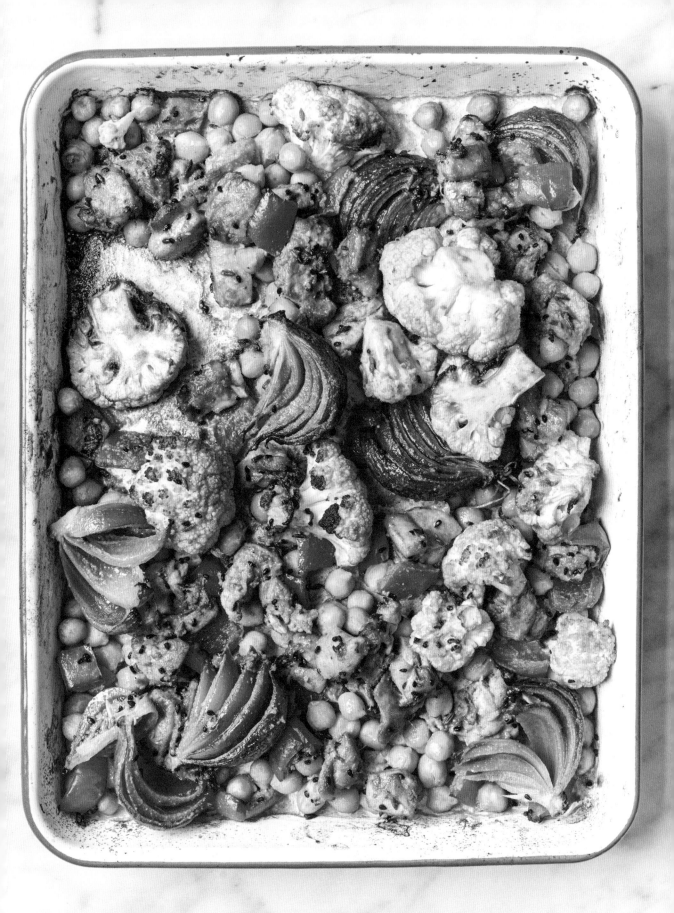

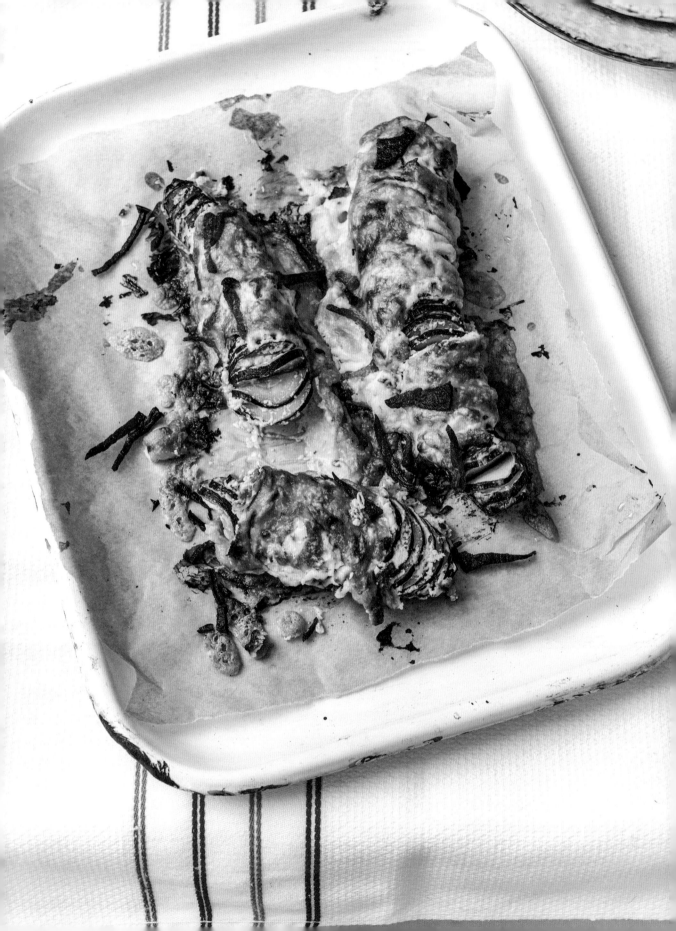

JALAPEÑO POPPER STUFFED COURGETTES

**SERVES 2 AS A MAIN,
4 AS A SIDE**
PREP TIME: 10 MINUTES
COOK TIME: 20 MINUTES

---

2 medium-sized courgettes
100g (3½oz) reduced-fat cream
    cheese
1 tablespoon very finely chopped
    pickled jalapeños
½ teaspoon garlic granules
½ teaspoon onion granules
2 smoked bacon medallions,
    cooked, then finely chopped
40g (1½oz) Cheddar cheese, grated
small handful of parsley leaves,
    finely chopped (optional)
salt and pepper

Make courgettes the star of a meal with this delicious twist on the famous jalapeño popper flavours. These can be a main course when served with rice and sweetcorn, or a delicious side dish. As a main course, serve one courgette per person (this recipe is easily doubled), or for a side dish allow half a courgette each.

1   Preheat the oven to 220°C/200°C fan (425°F), Gas Mark 7.

2   Slice off both ends of the courgettes, then line up chopsticks on either side of one of them. (If you don't have chopsticks, you could use 2 wooden spoon handles.) Carefully slice across the courgette from one end to the other in 5mm (¼ inch) thick slices, cutting down to the chopsticks to create a hasselback effect. Repeat with the other courgette.

3   Line a baking tray with nonstick baking paper, carefully transfer the courgettes to the baking paper and bake for 10 minutes.

4   Meanwhile, make the filling. In a bowl, mix the cream cheese, jalapeños, garlic and onion granules and salt and pepper.

5   Remove the courgettes from the oven (leave them on the baking tray) and use a table knife to ease a little bit of the cream cheese mixture between each slice, splitting it evenly between the courgettes. Scatter the bacon bits carefully over the top, then sprinkle with the Cheddar.

6   Bake for another 10 minutes, until the cheese is melted and golden brown. Scatter with parsley, if you like, then serve.

**PER SERVING
(AS A MAIN)**
CALORIES 250
FAT 15G
SAT FAT 8.5G
CARBS 6.2G
SUGARS 5.1G
FIBRE 3.7G
PROTEIN 21G
SALT 2.8G

Note

This delicious filling also works beautifully with hasselback baked potatoes or sweet potatoes. Simply slice in them in the same way as the courgettes here, bake them until soft, then add the filling and toppings and bake for 10 more minutes.

BACON, LEEK, POTATO & PEA BAKE

SERVES 4
PREP TIME: 15 MINUTES
COOK TIME: 55 MINUTES

spray oil

4 smoked bacon medallions, thinly
   sliced

1 large leek, or 2 medium leeks,
   trimmed, cleaned and finely
   chopped

4 garlic cloves, crushed

1 teaspoon dried thyme, plus more
   (optional) to serve

300ml (½ pint) hot chicken stock

100ml (3½fl oz) semi-skimmed
   milk

2 tablespoons white wine

800g (1lb 12oz) potatoes
   (5–6 large), peeled, halved
   lengthways and thinly sliced

300g (10½oz) frozen peas

120g (4¼oz) Cheddar cheese,
   grated

handful of parsley leaves, chopped,
   to serve (optional)

salt and pepper

When I first made this dish, I couldn't quite believe how delicious it was. The recipe was inspired by some sumptuous French favourites – tartiflette and boulangère potatoes – and I wanted that same indulgence and cheesy creaminess without overloading on calories. This hits the spot. It can easily be jazzed up with leftover ingredients such as ham, sausage, chorizo, chicken or mushrooms.

1   Preheat the oven to 200°C/180°C fan (400°F), Gas Mark 6.

2   Spray a frying pan with oil, place over a medium heat and fry the bacon and leek together for 5 minutes. Add the garlic and thyme, stir-fry for 30 seconds, then pour in the chicken stock, milk and wine. Stir everything to combine and season with salt and pepper.

3   Arrange half the sliced potatoes in a baking dish or shallow casserole dish, pour over half the leek mixture, then cover with a layer of all the frozen peas and half the Cheddar. Layer up the other half of the potatoes, then the remaining leek mixture and finally the rest of the Cheddar.

4   Put the lid on, or cover tightly with foil, and bake for 45 minutes until the potatoes are tender and cooked through. If the top needs a little further browning, grill it under a hot grill for a few minutes, then serve, scattered with chopped parsley or a sprinkle of dried thyme.

PER SERVING
CALORIES 438
FAT 14G
SAT FAT 7.4G
CARBS 46G
SUGARS 8.1G
FIBRE 9.1G
PROTEIN 26G
SALT 2.5G

Note

This is a dish where just a little amount of white wine really does add delicious flavour. It can be useful to have a mini bottle of wine on hand for recipes such as this which only require a small amount. Or many supermarkets now sell wine stock pots, so you can replace the chicken stock with wine stock, if you prefer.

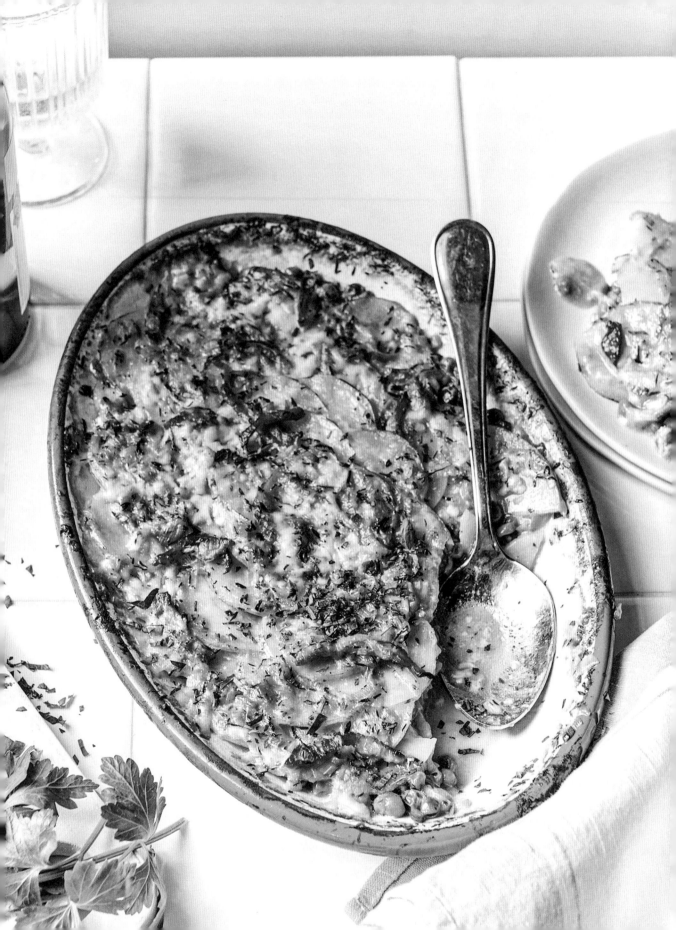

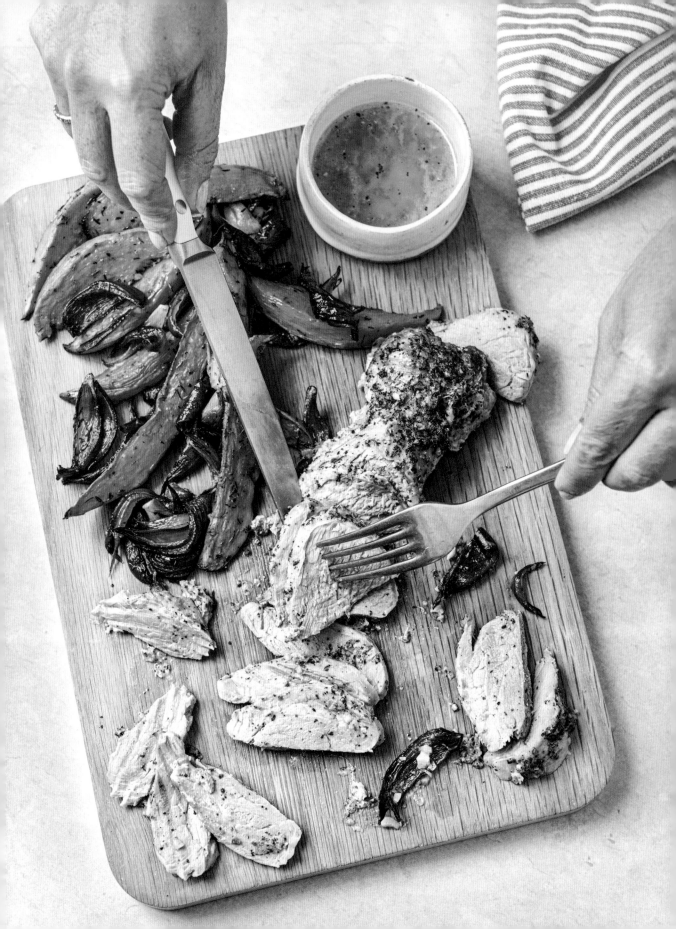

LEMON & GARLIC PORK WITH SWEET POTATO & ONION WEDGES

SERVES 4
PREP TIME: 10 MINUTES
COOK TIME: 35 MINUTES

1 tablespoon light mayonnaise
finely grated zest of 1 lemon
2 garlic cloves, crushed
1 teaspoon dried basil
1 teaspoon coarse ground salt
1 pork tenderloin/fillet (total
   weight 400–500g / 14oz–1lb 2oz)
2 medium-large sweet potatoes
   (total weight 750g / 1lb 10oz),
   peeled and cut into wedges
2 large red onions, cut into wedges
1 teaspoon dried thyme
freshly ground black pepper
spray oil, or low-calorie cooking
   spray

Pork tenderloin is a great cut for an easy and quick traybake, and using flavoured mayonnaise to coat it is a great way to keep it tender while cooking. Serve this with green vegetables such as broccoli, asparagus, green beans or peas.

1   Preheat the oven to 220°C/200°C fan (425°F), Gas Mark 7.

2   In a small bowl, mix the mayonnaise, lemon zest, garlic, basil and ½ teaspoon of the salt.

3   Make a foil 'boat' for the pork: fold a large piece of foil in half, place the pork in it, then turn up the edges all around to make a lip, so that the pork is nestled in it and the juices stay inside the foil. Place this in the middle of an extra-large baking tray and spread the mayonnaise mixture evenly over the pork (I use a teaspoon to do this).

4   Arrange the sweet potato and onion wedges around the pork in the tray, scatter over the thyme and the remaining ½ teaspoon of salt, grind on some pepper, then spray the wedges with spray oil, or low-calorie cooking spray. (If you don't have a baking tray large enough, simply use a separate tray for the pork and the wedges.)

5   Place the tray in the oven and bake for 30 minutes. Take the tray out of the oven, remove the pork to a chopping board to rest for a few minutes, then place the sweet potatoes and onion back in the oven for a final 5 minutes.

6   Slice the pork thinly and serve with the potatoes and onions, with some green veg of your choice on the side.

PER SERVING
CALORIES 406
FAT 4.8G
SAT FAT 2G
CARBS 46G
SUGARS 16G
FIBRE 5.6G
PROTEIN 42G
SALT 1.4G

Note

Try some different flavour combinations for the pork. Using the mayonnaise as a base, add a couple of teaspoons of different shop-bought spice mixes such as cajun, jerk or Mexican.

- ✓ SPAGHETTI FLORENTINE
- ✓ TANGY TAMARIND AND PRAWN WILD RICE
- ✓ CREAMY BASIL AND SUNDRIED TOMATO CHICKEN TAGLIATELLE
- ✓ STICKY HONEY-MUSTARD CHICKEN MUDDLE
- ✓ CHINESE 5-SPICE CHICKEN RICE
- ✓ TANDOORI CHICKEN BURGERS
- ✓ CHICKEN, PESTO AND PEA COUSCOUS
- ✓ ONE POT CHICKEN, LEMON AND ASPARAGUS FUSILLI
- ✓ SAUSAGE AND MUSHROOM RAGU
- ✓ BARBECUE BEEFARONI
- ✓ PHILLY CHEESESTEAK-STYLE ORZO
- ✓ TARRAGON CHICKEN AND MUSHROOM ORZO

3

Whip-It-Up Wednesday

SPAGHETTI FLORENTINE

SERVES 4
PREP TIME: 5 MINUTES
COOK TIME: 12 MINUTES

300g (10½oz) spaghetti

250g (9oz) ricotta cheese

1 teaspoon olive oil

30g (1oz) Parmesan-style
  vegetarian cheese, finely grated

finely grated zest and juice of
  1 lemon

1 garlic clove, crushed

½ teaspoon coarse ground salt

150g (5½oz) frozen spinach

freshly ground black pepper

handful of herb leaves, such as
  parsley or basil, to serve

A simple, delicious pasta which harnesses the classic combination of ricotta and spinach, with a hint of lemon. This is delicious all year round but especially suits warm summer evenings. Serve it with a simple rocket salad.

1   Cook the spaghetti according to the packet instructions in a large pan of boiling water.

2   Meanwhile, in a bowl, mix together the ricotta, olive oil, Parmesan-style cheese, lemon zest and juice, garlic and salt. Add a ladle of the hot pasta water to loosen the mixture and help you stir it into a smooth sauce.

3   For the last 2 minutes of the spaghetti cooking time, add the frozen spinach to the pan and stir to defrost it. Drain the spaghetti and spinach, reserving a little more of the cooking water.

4   Stir the ricotta sauce into the spaghetti, loosening it with the reserved pasta water if it isn't saucy enough.

5   Divide between 4 pasta bowls and add freshly ground black pepper and a sprinkling of fresh herbs.

PER SERVING
CALORIES 411
FAT 13G
SAT FAT 7.1G
CARBS 54G
SUGARS 4.6G
FIBRE 5G
PROTEIN 18G
SALT 0.98G

Note

Bacon pieces, or finely chopped chorizo, work well in this dish. Simply fry them separately and stir into the sauce with the spaghetti.

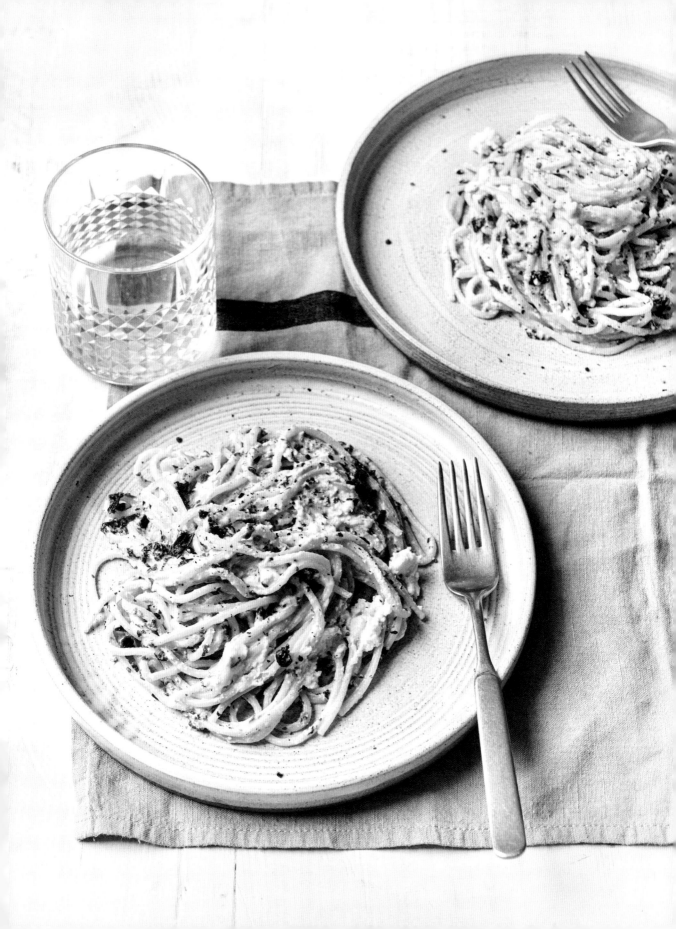

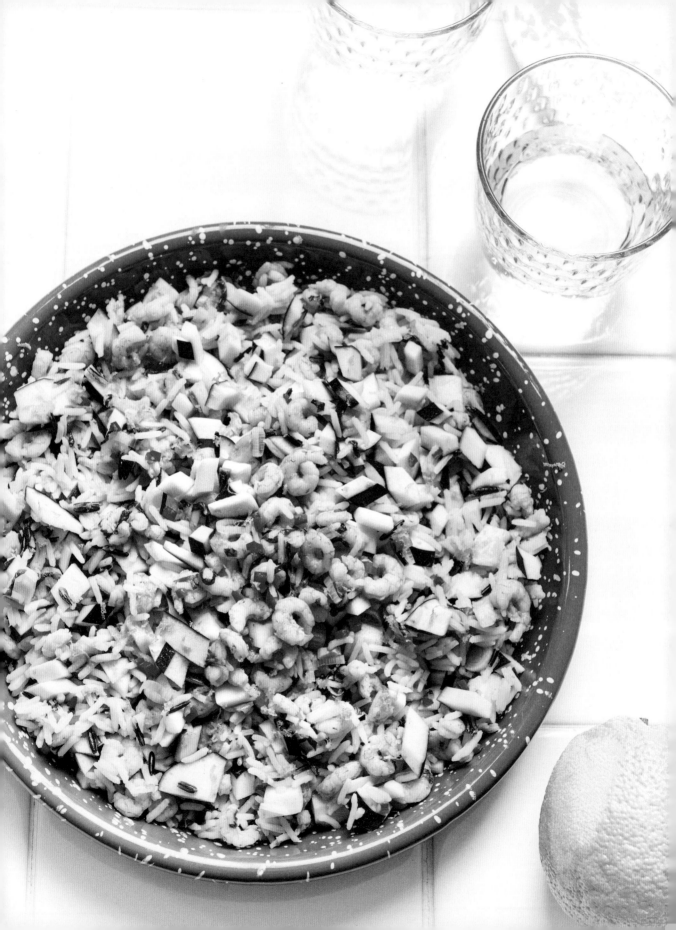

TANGY TAMARIND & PRAWN WILD RICE

SERVES 4
PREP TIME: 10 MINUTES
COOK TIME: 20 MINUTES

300g (10½oz) cooked and peeled cold-water prawns, defrosted if frozen

1 tablespoon maple syrup

1 tablespoon fish sauce

2 garlic cloves, crushed

2 teaspoons tamarind paste

1 red chilli, deseeded and finely chopped

finely grated zest and juice of 1 orange

6 spring onions, finely sliced

large handful of basil leaves, shredded, plus more to serve

1 teaspoon coarse ground salt

280g (10oz) mixed basmati and wild rice (or see recipe introduction)

1 tablespoon sesame oil

1 large courgette, finely chopped

freshly ground black pepper

There is plenty of flavour packed into this simple rice dish. I use mixed rice because it looks and tastes more interesting – the wild rice has more of a chewy texture, which adds some variety – but you can use just basmati or jasmine rice if you can't find wild rice.

1   Put the defrosted prawns in a bowl and add the maple syrup, fish sauce, garlic, tamarind paste, chilli, most of the orange zest (reserve a little), all the orange juice, the spring onions, basil and salt. Mix and leave to marinate.

2   Put the rice on to cook, according to the packet instructions.

3   When the rice has 5 minutes left, heat the sesame oil in a sauté pan and, once it's hot, add the prawns and all the marinade and stir-fry for 5 minutes.

4   Drain the rice, then add the courgette and the prawns and mix everything together thoroughly.

5   Serve sprinkled with the remaining orange zest, a little more basil and a few grinds of black pepper.

PER SERVING
CALORIES 372
FAT 4.8G
SAT FAT 0.8G
CARBS 61G
SUGARS 6.5G
FIBRE 2.5G
PROTEIN 20G
SALT 3.3G

Note

I like the crunch of raw courgette in this, but if you would prefer it to be softer, then fry it along with the prawns and their marinade. You could also add some crunchy finely chopped peppers at the end, instead of or as well as the courgette.

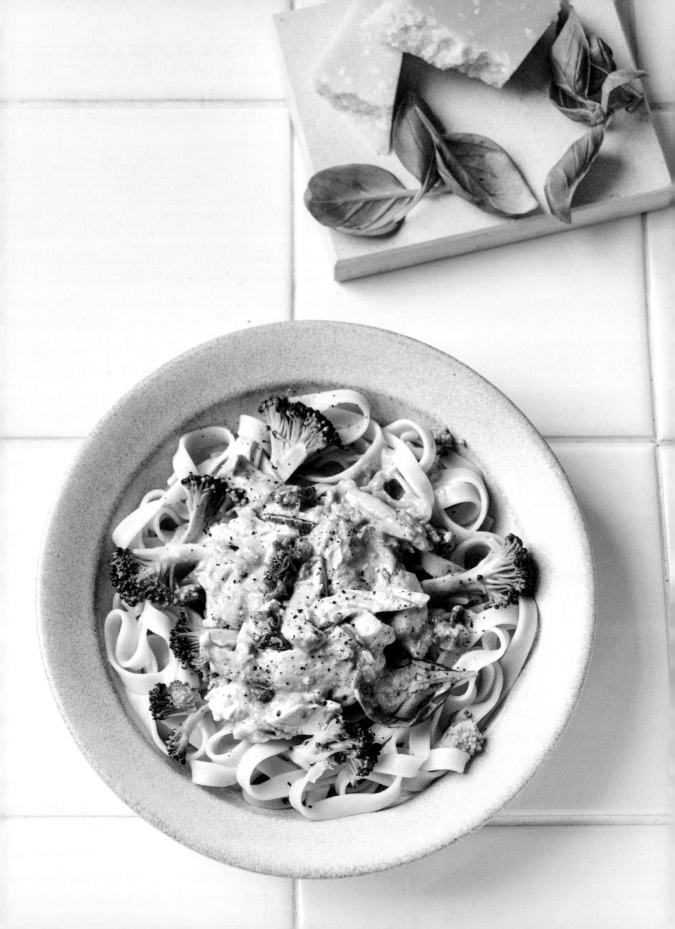

CREAMY BASIL & SUNDRIED TOMATO CHICKEN TAGLIATELLE

SERVES 4
PREP TIME: 10 MINUTES
COOK TIME: 20 MINUTES

spray oil

4 shallots, finely chopped

3 chicken breasts (total weight about 500g / 1lb 2oz), finely sliced

2 large garlic cloves, crushed

50g (1¾oz) sundried tomatoes, drained and finely chopped

300ml (½ pint) hot chicken stock

300g (10½oz) tagliatelle (or see recipe introduction)

1 head of broccoli, broken up into florets

100g (3½oz) reduced-fat cream cheese

salt and pepper

large handful of basil leaves (about 10g / ¼oz), shredded, plus more to serve

Parmesan cheese, finely grated, to serve (optional)

In my household, this meal always results in clean bowls all round. The recipe works well with long pasta such as tagliatelle, linguine or spaghetti, because the creamy sauce coats and clings to the strands, but you can use any pasta shape you have in. The sauce also pairs brilliantly with a mixed leaf salad.

1   Spray a sauté pan or deep frying pan with oil, place over a medium heat and add the shallots, sliced chicken, garlic and sundried tomatoes. Stir-fry for 5 minutes.

2   Pour in the chicken stock and simmer for 10 minutes.

3   Meanwhile, put the tagliatelle in a large pan of boiling water and cook according to the packet instructions. Either pop the broccoli into a separate medium pan of boiling water towards the end of the pasta cooking time and simmer for 3–4 minutes, or just add it with the pasta for the last 3–4 minutes of cooking time to save using another pan.

4   Stir the cream cheese into the chicken sauce and simmer gently for a couple more minutes while you drain the pasta and broccoli. Season the creamy sauce to taste with salt and pepper and stir in the basil.

5   Divide the pasta and broccoli between 4 pasta bowls and serve the creamy chicken sauce over the top. Sprinkle with some more basil and Parmesan, if using, then serve.

Note

PER SERVING
CALORIES 555
FAT 13G
SAT FAT 3.5G
CARBS 57G
SUGARS 6.4G
FIBRE 9.9G
PROTEIN 47G
SALT 1.4G

> This sauce is a great way to use up bits and bobs of extra vegetables that you have in the refrigerator or freezer: you can fry sliced mushrooms, leeks or celery in step 1, or add quick-cooking green vegetables such as green beans, peas, broad beans or asparagus about 5 minutes into step 2. If you have a bottle of white wine open, then a good glug stirred through just before you pour in the chicken stock will add delicious flavour.

> For a vegetarian version, leave out the chicken and use mushrooms instead, swap the chicken stock for vegetable stock, and use a Parmesan-style vegetarian cheese instead of Parmesan.

> For a lighter option, serve the sauce over courgetti instead of tagliatelle.

STICKY HONEY-MUSTARD CHICKEN MUDDLE

SERVES 4
PREP TIME: 15 MINUTES
COOK TIME: 25 MINUTES

500g (1lb 2oz) baby potatoes, halved, or quartered if large

spray oil

6 skinless chicken thigh fillets

1 red onion, chopped

½ pointed spring cabbage, shredded

250ml (9fl oz) hot chicken stock

2 tablespoons honey

2 tablespoons wholegrain mustard

1 tablespoon red wine vinegar

1 teaspoon paprika

1 teaspoon Italian-style mixed herbs

1 teaspoon coarse ground salt

4 spring onions, finely sliced (optional)

freshly ground black pepper

Shredded chicken thighs, new potatoes and tender cabbage come together in a rich honey-mustard glaze for this simple all-in-one dish.

1   Put the potatoes into a pan of simmering water and leave them simmering for 15 minutes. Meanwhile, start to cook the other ingredients.

2   Spray a sauté pan with spray oil and place over a medium heat. Add the chicken thigh fillets and onion, then fry for 10 minutes, turning the chicken over halfway.

3   Add the cabbage, then stir-fry for another 5 minutes.

4   Drain the potatoes, tip them into the sauté pan, then pour in the chicken stock and add the honey, mustard, red wine vinegar, paprika, mixed herbs and salt. Bring up to a simmer and cook for 10 minutes, stirring regularly.

5   Remove the cooked chicken from the pan, slice it thinly, then return it to the pan. Scatter with the spring onions, if using, grind over some pepper, then serve.

PER SERVING
CALORIES 347
FAT 3.7G
SAT FAT 1.7G
CARBS 28G
SUGARS 11G
FIBRE 4.1G
PROTEIN 49G
SALT 2.2G

Note

For an even quicker version, use canned new potatoes to eliminate the step of boiling the potatoes.

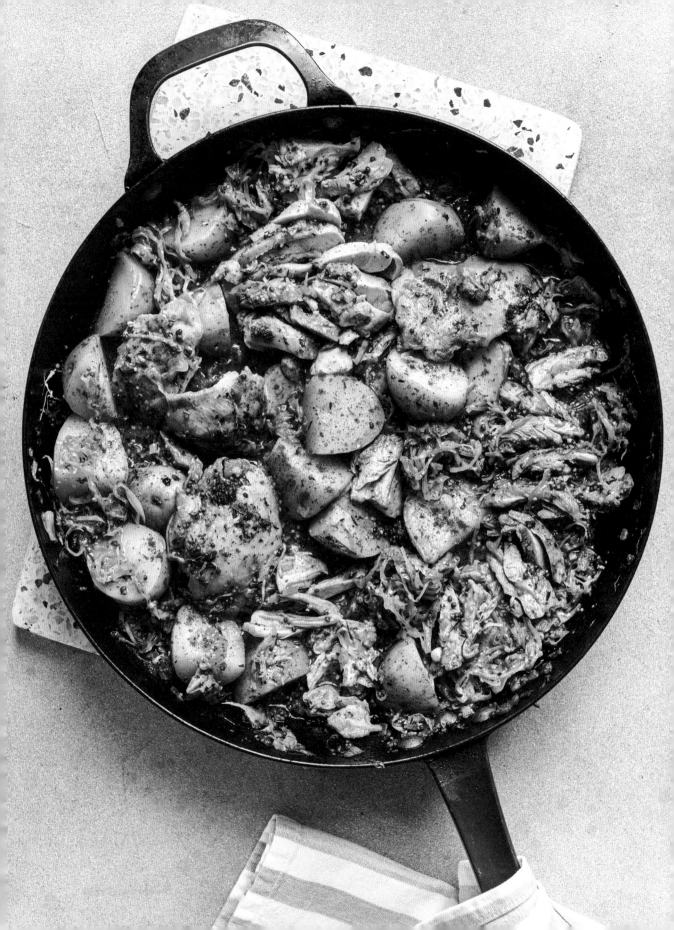

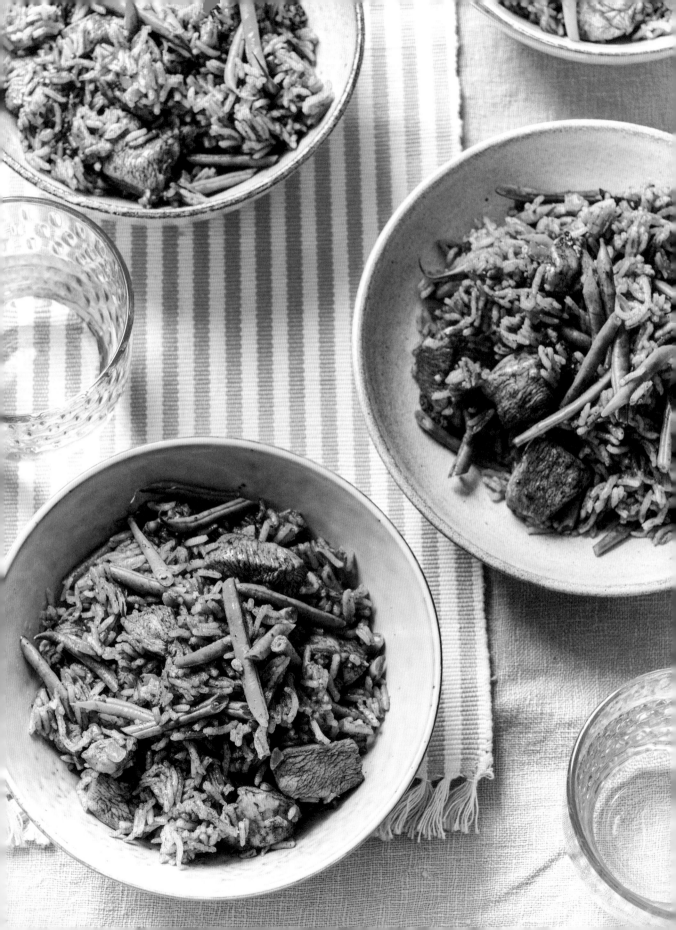

CHINESE 5-SPICE CHICKEN RICE

SERVES 4
PREP TIME: 10 MINUTES
COOK TIME: 20 MINUTES

1 red onion, finely chopped

2 tablespoons Shaoxing rice wine

2 tablespoons dark soy sauce

1 tablespoon tomato purée

1 tablespoon Chinese 5-spice

2 garlic cloves, crushed

3 skinless chicken breasts, chopped into small pieces

spray oil

200g (7oz) basmati rice

450ml (16fl oz) hot chicken stock

200g (7oz) fine green beans, topped and tailed and cut into 1cm (½ inch) pieces

This is everything you want from a Whip-It-Up Wednesday recipe: an easy and quick, family-friendly one-pot meal.

1 Put the red onion, rice wine, soy sauce, tomato purée, Chinese 5-spice and garlic into a medium-sized bowl and mix it all together. Add the chicken and stir to thoroughly coat.

2 Spray oil on to a sauté pan or casserole dish which has a lid, place over a high heat, then add the chicken and sauce and stir-fry for 5 minutes.

3 Stir in the rice, then pour in the stock, cover with the lid and simmer gently for 15 minutes, stirring halfway to ensure nothing is sticking to the bottom of the pan.

4 Add the green beans, stir again, replace the lid and leave to rest for 10 minutes with the heat off. After this time, the rice should be tender and the beans will retain a bit of crunch.

PER SERVING
CALORIES 370
FAT 2.5G
SAT FAT 0.6G
CARBS 48G
SUGARS 7.7G
FIBRE 3.1G
PROTEIN 36G
SALT 1.9G

Note

For a vegetarian alternative, replace the chicken with 350g (12oz) chestnut mushrooms cut into quarters, or button mushrooms, left whole.

TANDOORI CHICKEN BURGERS

SERVES 4
PREP TIME: 15 MINUTES
COOK TIME: 14 MINUTES

Tender spiced chicken burgers – served in flatbreads with carrot salad and lemon and mint yogurt sauce – are a great, light and flavoursome alternative to traditional burgers.

500g (1lb 2oz) lean minced chicken (less than 5 per cent fat)

2 spring onions, finely sliced

3cm (1¼ inch) piece of fresh root ginger, peeled and finely grated

1½ tablespoons mild tandoori powder

1 tablespoon oats (not jumbo)

½ teaspoon coarse ground salt

4 folded flatbreads (white, wholemeal or seeded)

4 teaspoons mango chutney

FOR THE CARROT SALAD

4 medium carrots (total weight about 400g / 14oz), grated

1 red chilli, finely chopped

1 teaspoon nigella seeds

juice of 1 small lemon (zest it first, for the sauce)

FOR THE LEMON AND MINT SAUCE

120g (4¼oz) fat-free Greek yogurt

small handful of mint leaves, finely chopped

finely grated zest of 1 lemon (from the lemon in the salad)

1   In a medium-sized bowl, mix the chicken, spring onions, ginger, tandoori powder, oats and salt until well combined. The best way is to use your hands, to make sure that all the ingredients are evenly distributed. Form the mixture into 4 equally sized burger patties.

2   Make the carrot salad by simply mixing all the ingredients together in a bowl with a pinch of salt.

3   For the sauce, again mix the ingredients together in a small bowl with another pinch of salt.

4   Preheat the grill to high. Line a baking tray with foil and lay the burgers on the foil. Press into the middle of each burger with your thumb to create an indent (this helps it to cook evenly).

5   Grill the burgers for 12–14 minutes, flipping them carefully with a spatula every few minutes, until they are golden brown and cooked through.

6   Pop the flatbreads in a toaster for about 1 minute, just to warm them through and very lightly toast them.

7   Spread the bottom inside half of each flatbread with mango chutney, add a couple of spoons of carrot salad, lay a burger on, then add a spoonful of lemon and mint sauce on top. Serve immediately.

PER SERVING
CALORIES 358
FAT 8.2G
SAT FAT 1.7G
CARBS 35G
SUGARS 14G
FIBRE 7.6G
PROTEIN 32G
SALT 1.9G

Note

If you can't get hold of minced chicken, then minced turkey also works well in these.

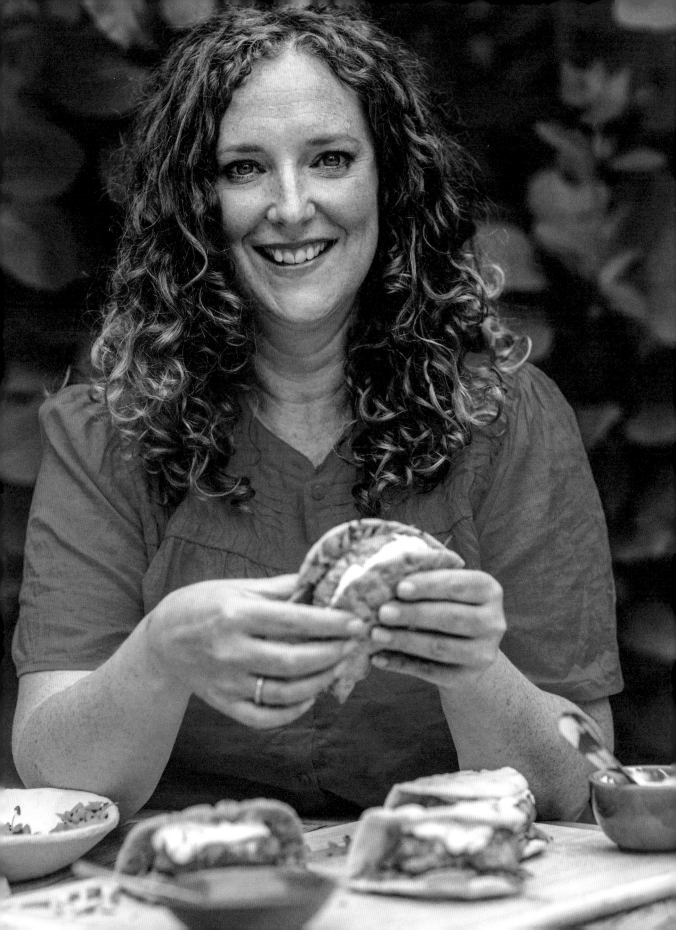

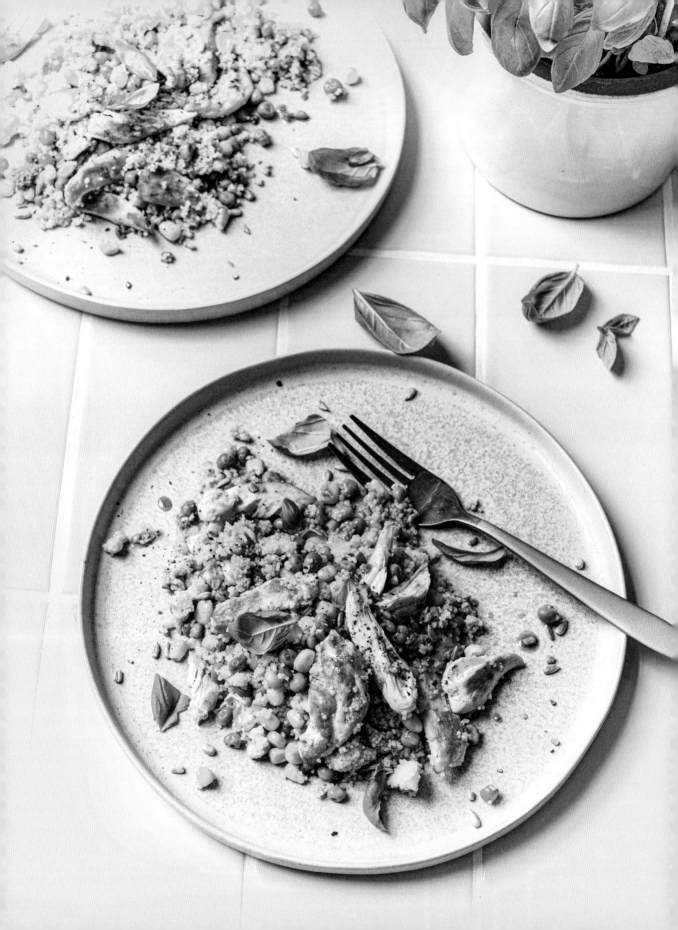

CHICKEN, PESTO & PEA COUSCOUS

SERVES 4
PREP TIME: 5 MINUTES
COOK TIME: 15 MINUTES

spray oil

2 large skinless chicken breasts
(total weight about 400g / 14oz),
halved lengthways and finely
sliced

200g (7oz) wholewheat couscous

300ml (½ pint) boiling hot chicken
stock

40g (1½oz) sunflower seeds

finely grated zest and juice of
1 lemon

125g (4½oz) frozen petits pois

125g (4½oz) frozen sweetcorn

3 tablespoons green pesto

salt and pepper

torn basil leaves, or chopped
parsley leaves, to serve

There aren't many meals you can get on the table in 20 minutes, so this recipe is a great weapon to have in your arsenal for days when you really don't have time to spare. Pesto-coated chicken and couscous with a zing of lemon and some crunch from the sweetcorn and sunflower seeds, this is delicious hot and cold, making it perfect picnic and lunchbox food as well as a satisfying dinner.

1   Spray a sauté pan with oil and place over a medium heat. Add the chicken to the pan and fry for about 12 minutes, stirring occasionally.

2   Once you've put the chicken on, pour the measured couscous into a bowl, pour over the hot chicken stock and place a plate over the top to cover.

3   Put the sunflower seeds into a dry frying pan over a high heat and toast them for 2 minutes, then remove from the heat and set aside.

4   After 12 minutes, check that there is no pink left inside the thickest part of the chicken, season it with salt and pepper, then stir in the lemon zest and juice, then the frozen petits pois and sweetcorn. Stir-fry for 2 minutes.

5   Fluff up the couscous with a fork, then add it to the pan with the chicken, reducing the heat to low. Spoon in the pesto and stir it through until fully distributed. Sprinkle the sunflower seeds over with some herbs, then serve.

PER SERVING
CALORIES 468
FAT 15G
SAT FAT 3.1G
CARBS 41G
SUGARS 4.8G
FIBRE 8.6G
PROTEIN 38G
SALT 0.92G

Note

Try variations on this recipe using different flavours of pesto, or for a vegetarian option, use vegetarian-friendly pesto and vegetable stock and replace the chicken with cubes of vegetarian halloumi, which will take about 6 minutes to fry in step 1.

ONE-POT CHICKEN, LEMON & ASPARAGUS FUSILLI

SERVES 4
PREP TIME: 10 MINUTES
COOK TIME: 30 MINUTES

---

spray oil

2 large skinless chicken breasts (total weight about 400g / 14oz), finely chopped

3 garlic cloves, crushed

600ml (1 pint) hot chicken stock

300g (10½oz) fusilli

½ teaspoon dried oregano

250g (9oz) asparagus spears, trimmed and sliced into pieces

finely grated zest and juice of 1 lemon

salt and pepper

Parmesan shavings, to serve (optional)

It's always good to have a simple pasta dish in your kitchen repertoire for busy evenings, and this light, fresh dish is great for feeding the family. I was surprised that my slightly fussy girls would go for asparagus, but they happily eat it in this, where it's cut up into manageable bite-sized pieces. If asparagus is not in season, feel free to swap it out for fine green beans, sugar snaps, broccoli or runner beans.

1   Spray a large saucepan or sauté pan, which has a lid, with oil and place over a medium heat. Fry the chicken for 5 minutes and season with salt and pepper. Stir the garlic through and cook for 1 minute, then pour in the chicken stock and add the fusilli and oregano.

2   Bring to the boil, then stir, reduce the heat to a simmer, put the lid on the pan and simmer gently for 15 minutes.

3   Add the asparagus, place the lid back on and cook gently for 5 more minutes.

4   Stir the lemon zest and juice through the pasta and serve, with Parmesan shavings, if you like.

PER SERVING
CALORIES 468
FAT 15G
SAT FAT 3.1G
CARBS 41G
SUGARS 4.8G
FIBRE 8.6G
PROTEIN 38G
SALT 0.92G

Note

For a vegetarian version, leave out the chicken, replace the chicken stock with vegetable stock and add extra fresh green vegetables in at the same time as the asparagus: try chopped courgettes, green beans, broccoli, runner beans or peas. Substitute the Parmesan for a Parmesan-style vegetarian cheese.

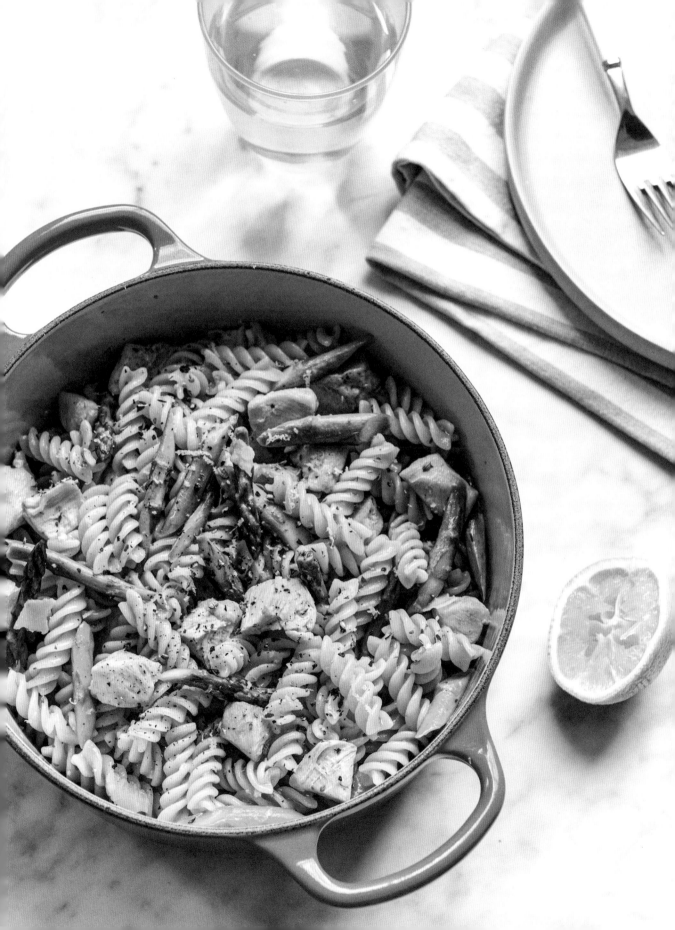

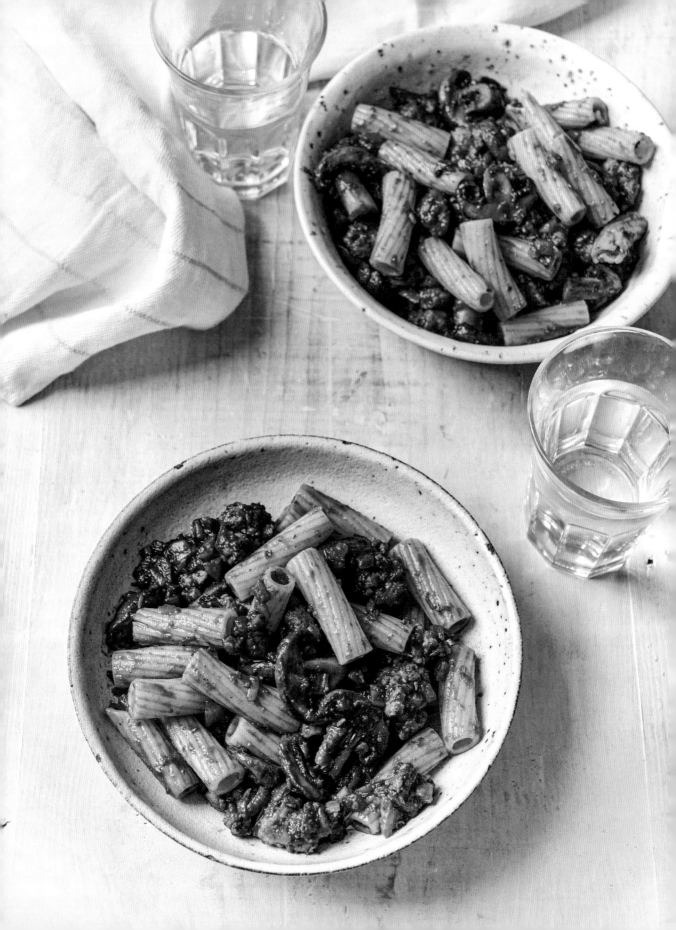

SAUSAGE & MUSHROOM RAGU

SERVES 4
PREP TIME: 12 MINUTES
COOK TIME: 35 MINUTES

spray oil

1 onion, finely chopped

2 celery stalks, finely chopped

1 medium carrot, grated

3 garlic cloves, crushed

250g (9oz) chestnut mushrooms, sliced

1 teaspoon fennel seeds (see note below)

1 teaspoon dried oregano

1 teaspoon dried rosemary, or finely chopped fresh rosemary leaves

400g (14oz) reduced-fat pork sausages, squeezed out of their skins, or finely chopped if the meat doesn't easily come out of the skins (about 6-8 sausages)

4 tablespoons balsamic vinegar

300g (10½oz) tomato passata

200ml (7fl oz) water

300g (10½oz) pasta (tagliatelle, pappardelle and rigatoni all work well)

salt and pepper

Parmesan cheese, finely grated, to serve (optional)

Sausages are a wonderfully convenient way to get quick flavour into meals, and now that most supermarkets sell reduced-fat sausages, you can make a healthy meal with them. This is like a Bolognese sauce, though the fennel and sausage provide a different flavour twist.

1   Spray a sauté pan with oil, set it over a medium heat and stir-fry the onion, celery, carrot, garlic, mushrooms and fennel seeds for 8 minutes.

2   Stir in the oregano and rosemary, then add the sausagemeat, or chopped sausages, and stir-fry for 5 minutes until the meat is browned.

3   Stir the balsamic vinegar through, then pour in the passata and water. Season with salt and pepper and allow to simmer for 20 minutes, stirring occasionally, until the sauce is reduced and not watery.

4   Meanwhile, cook the pasta according to the packet instructions, then drain.

5   Stir the pasta through the ragu to coat, then serve.

PER SERVING
CALORIES 376
FAT 10G
SAT FAT 3.2G
CARBS 48G
SUGARS 9.6G
FIBRE 6G
PROTEIN 20G
SALT 1.2G

Note

> Fennel has a strong and distinctive flavour. If you're making this sauce for kids for the first time, you may wish to reduce the amount of fennel to ½ teaspoon, just to introduce them to the flavour. You can also customize the sauce as you wish: I love fresh chilli added when I'm frying everything in step 1, while a glug of red wine added at the same time as the passata in step 3 gives delicious flavour.

> You can freeze the sauce but not the pasta.

BARBECUE BEEFARONI

SERVES 4
PREP TIME: 10 MINUTES
COOK TIME: 30 MINUTES

spray oil

1 onion, chopped

3 smoked bacon medallions, thinly sliced

150g (5½oz) cherry tomatoes, halved

1 red pepper, deseeded and chopped

2 garlic cloves, crushed

250g (9oz) lean minced beef (less than 5 per cent fat)

1 litre (1¾ pints) hot beef stock

300g (10½oz) macaroni

150ml (¼ pint) tomato passata

2 tablespoons balsamic vinegar

2 tablespoons tomato purée

1 tablespoon Worcestershire sauce

1 tablespoon honey

2 teaspoons dried oregano

½ teaspoon smoked paprika

1 teaspoon coarse ground salt

60g (2¼oz) red Leicester cheese, grated

I spotted a tin of 'beefaroni' on an American TV show and I was curious… it turns out it's canned pasta with a minced beef and tomato sauce. I loved this idea and decided to add a barbecue flavour twist to this homemade version. It's relaxed one-pot cooking and a great crowd-pleasing recipe. Plus it only uses half a standard pack of minced beef, so you can get another meal out of it (such as my Beef and Black Bean Burgers with Hot Corn Salsa, see page 131).

1 Spray a large, deep saucepan with oil, place over a medium heat and fry the onion and bacon for 5 minutes. Add the cherry tomatoes, red pepper and garlic and fry for 5 more minutes, stirring every now and again. Add the minced beef, then stir-fry for a few minutes to brown it and break up any clumps.

2 Pour in the beef stock and add the macaroni, passata, balsamic vinegar, tomato purée, Worcestershire sauce, honey, oregano, paprika and salt, stir well, then leave simmering for 15 minutes, stirring occasionally. The macaroni should be cooked through and the sauce thick, not watery. If it's still a little watery, increase the heat and give it a good bubble for a couple of minutes to boil away the excess liquid.

3 Add the cheese to the pot and stir through before serving.

PER SERVING
CALORIES 539
FAT 12G
SAT FAT 5.2G
CARBS 64G
SUGARS 14G
FIBRE 8G
PROTEIN 37G
SALT 4.1G

Note

This is also great with beans: try adding a can of borlotti, pinto or kidney beans (drained and rinsed) to simmer with everything in step 2.

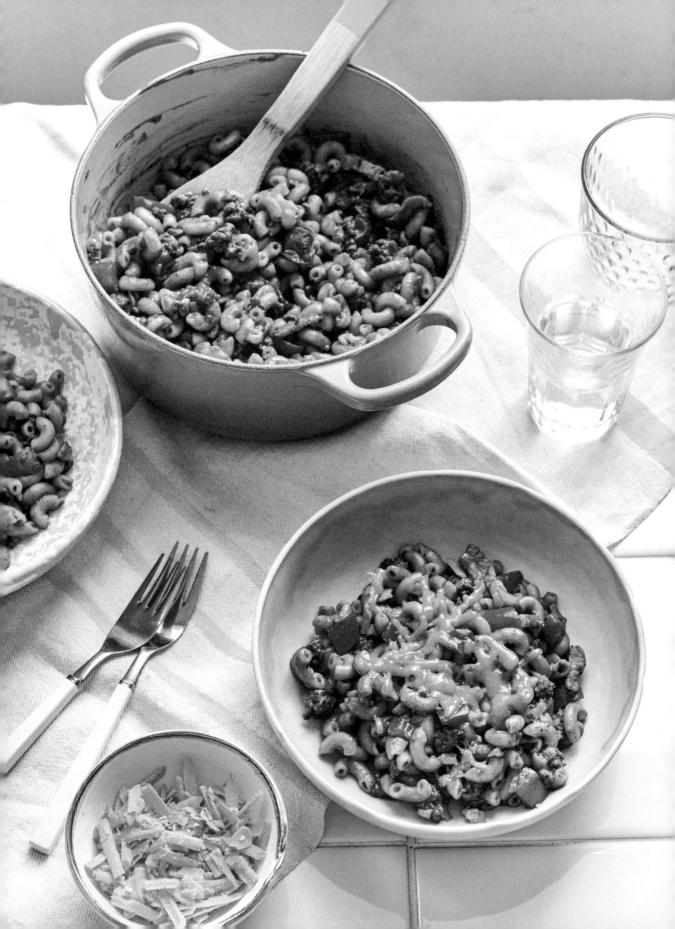

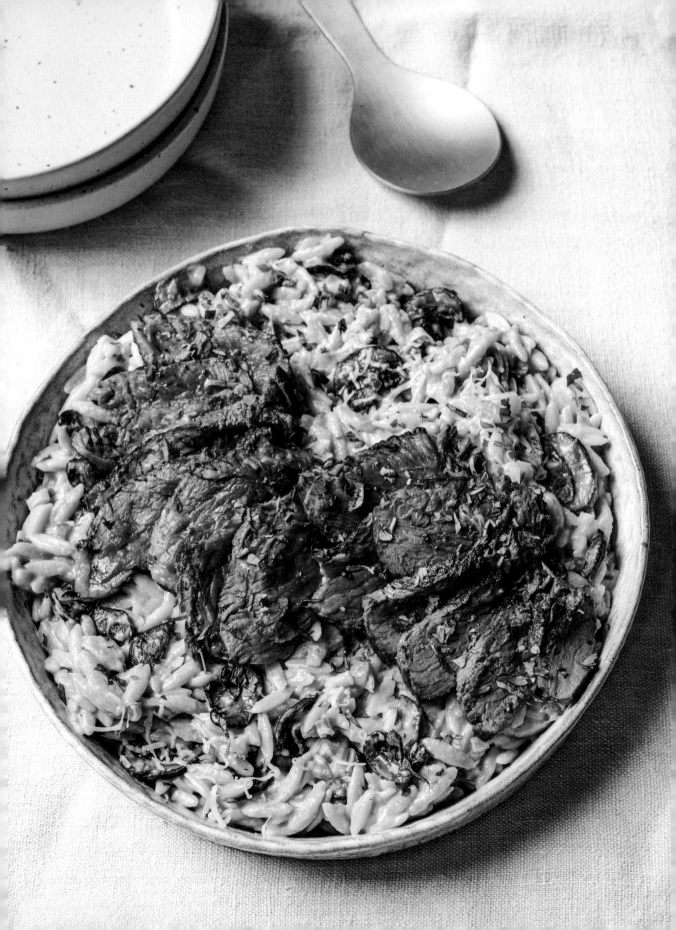

PHILLY CHEESESTEAK-STYLE ORZO

SERVES 4
PREP TIME: 10 MINUTES
COOK TIME: 12 MINUTES

360g (12½oz) orzo

spray oil

2 rump steaks (total weight about 450g / 1lb), at room temperature

1 onion, chopped

1 green pepper, deseeded and chopped

250g (9oz) chestnut mushrooms, sliced

75g (2¾oz) reduced-fat cream cheese

60g (2¼oz) Cheddar cheese, grated

salt and pepper

handful of parsley leaves, chopped, to serve

FOR THE SAUCE

1 tablespoon Worcestershire sauce

1 tablespoon soy sauce

1 teaspoon garlic granules

½ teaspoon onion granules

¼ teaspoon mustard powder

finely chopped parsley leaves, to serve

PER SERVING
CALORIES 596
FAT 14G
SAT FAT 6.8G
CARBS 74G
SUGARS 6.1G
FIBRE 3.7G
PROTEIN 46G
SALT 1.5G

You can't beat the flavours in a Philly cheesesteak, so I've borrowed them for this quick but luxurious orzo dish.

1   Make up the sauce by mixing all the ingredients together in a small bowl.

2   Put the orzo on to cook following the packet instructions (usually 8–10 minutes).

3   Spray a frying pan with oil and fry the steak according to your preference (see note below). Set the steak aside to rest on a plate.

4   Add the onion and pepper to the frying pan. Stir-fry these for 5 minutes, then add the mushrooms and stir-fry for another 3 minutes. Pour the sauce into the frying pan with the vegetables and stir through.

5   Drain the orzo, reserving a little of the cooking water, and add it to the vegetables, with the cream cheese and Cheddar, a little of the reserved pasta cooking water and some salt and pepper. Stir together thoroughly.

6   Thinly slice the steak with a sharp knife and season with salt and pepper.

7   Divide the orzo between 4 bowls, top with the strips of steak and scatter with parsley before serving.

Note

Allowing steak to reach room temperature before cooking will help it to cook evenly. The thickness of your steak will affect its cooking time. As a general rule of thumb, for a steak around 2cm (¾ inch) thick:

> for rare, cook for 3 minutes, turning halfway through

> for medium-rare, cook for 4 minutes, turning halfway through

> for medium, cook for 4½ minutes, turning halfway through

> for well done, cook for 8 minutes, turning halfway through

Leaving steak to rest for at least 5 minutes after cooking will allow it to reabsorb its juices, so it isn't tough.

TARRAGON CHICKEN & MUSHROOM ORZO

SERVES 4
PREP TIME: 10 MINUTES
COOK TIME: 35 MINUTES

spray oil

1 onion, chopped

2 skinless chicken breasts, cut into small bite-sized pieces

200g (7oz) chestnut mushrooms, sliced

50ml (2fl oz) white wine

300g (10½oz) orzo

1 litre (1¾ pints) hot chicken stock

2 teaspoons Dijon mustard

150g (5½oz) frozen spinach

1 tablespoon finely chopped tarragon leaves

50g (1¾oz) reduced-fat crème fraîche

salt and pepper

There is something very satisfying about the flavour of fresh tarragon: it has a light, delicate liquorice-y taste, but with far more complexity. There's a magic about its savouriness which has me craving it again as soon as I've eaten it, thinking I should cook with it more often. This is a tasty, easy, one-pot dish.

1   Spray a sauté pan with oil and place over a medium-high heat. Fry the onion for a few minutes, then add the chicken and mushrooms and stir-fry for about 10 minutes.

2   Pour in the white wine, bring to the boil and simmer for 1 minute, then stir through the orzo. Pour in three-quarters of the chicken stock, add the mustard and simmer for 15 minutes, stirring occasionally.

3   Now add the spinach and pour in the remaining stock, stir well and simmer for another 5 minutes.

4   Add the tarragon and crème fraîche, season to taste with salt and pepper, stir well to ensure the crème fraîche has melted and the spinach and tarragon are well distributed, then serve.

PER SERVING
CALORIES 483
FAT 6.2G
SAT FAT 2.2G
CARBS 60G
SUGARS 8G
FIBRE 7.5G
PROTEIN 41G
SALT 2G

Note

Not all supermarkets sell fresh tarragon, but the larger ones do. If you can't get hold of it, you could replace it in this dish with basil leaves, fennel fronds, dill, or simply a tablespoon of pesto.

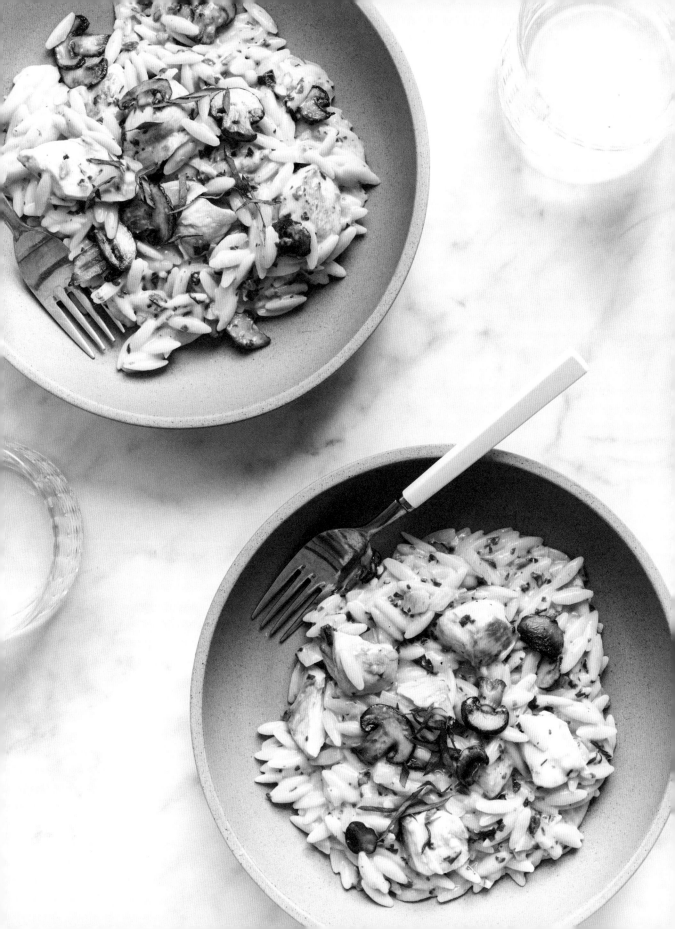

- ✓ SPAGHETTI FRITTATA
- ✓ PASTA SAUCES 3 WAYS
- ✓ BLACK BEAN, KALE AND SWEET POTATO CURRY
- ✓ COURGETTE PESTO PASTA
- ✓ MEDITERRANEAN-STYLE TUNA AND VEGETABLE CRUMBLE
- ✓ TUNA AND LEEK PASTA BAKE
- ✓ SOUL-FOOD SWEET POTATO AND CHICKEN SOUP
- ✓ CRUNCHY VIETNAMESE-STYLE CHICKEN SALAD
- ✓ PARMIGIANA DI MELANZANE
- ✓ FRENCH ONION ORZOTTO
- ✓ SIMPLE RED LENTIL DAL

4

Thrifty Thursday

SPAGHETTI FRITTATA

SERVES 4
PREP TIME: 5 MINUTES
COOK TIME: 35 MINUTES

200g (7oz) spaghetti

6 eggs

30g (1oz) Parmesan-style vegetarian cheese, finely grated

1 teaspoon dried parsley

1 teaspoon dried basil

spray oil

2 shallots, halved and thinly sliced

4 large handfuls of chopped kale, coarse stalks removed

2 garlic cloves, crushed

200g (7oz) tomato passata

100g (3½oz) mozzarella cheese

salt and pepper

herb leaves, such as parsley or basil, to serve (optional)

An extra-filling frittata which is delicious hot or cold. Perfect for picnics, packed lunches, or served up with salad at mealtimes.

1. Preheat the oven to 200°C/180°C fan (400°F), Gas Mark 6.

2. Cook the spaghetti according to the packet instructions. Meanwhile, prepare the other ingredients.

3. Lightly beat the eggs with the Parmesan, parsley, basil and some salt and pepper.

4. Spray a large frying pan with oil and sauté the shallots for 2 minutes. Add the kale and stir-fry for another 5 minutes, then stir through the garlic.

5. Drain the spaghetti, add it to the frying pan, pour in the passata, season with a little more salt and pepper and stir to combine evenly.

6. Line a round or square baking dish (I use a round 24cm / 9½ inch baking dish) with nonstick baking paper. Decant the spaghetti into the baking dish, make sure it is evenly spread, then pour over the egg mixture, tipping the dish from side to side to spread it as evenly as possible. Break up the mozzarella into small pieces and dot all over the top.

7. Place on the middle shelf of the oven and bake for 25 minutes, until the top is golden brown and the eggs solid all the way through. (If you used a different-sized dish, you may need to slightly adjust the cooking time: in a large dish the frittata will be shallower and so will cook more quickly.) Scatter with fresh herb, if using, then slice and serve.

PER SERVING
CALORIES 423
FAT 17G
SAT FAT 7.2G
CARBS 39G
SUGARS 5.4G
FIBRE 4.3G
PROTEIN 26G
SALT 1G

Note

You can add pizza-style toppings to this if you like: anchovies, olives, different cheeses, chorizo, mushrooms, artichoke hearts, peppers and tomatoes will all work well.

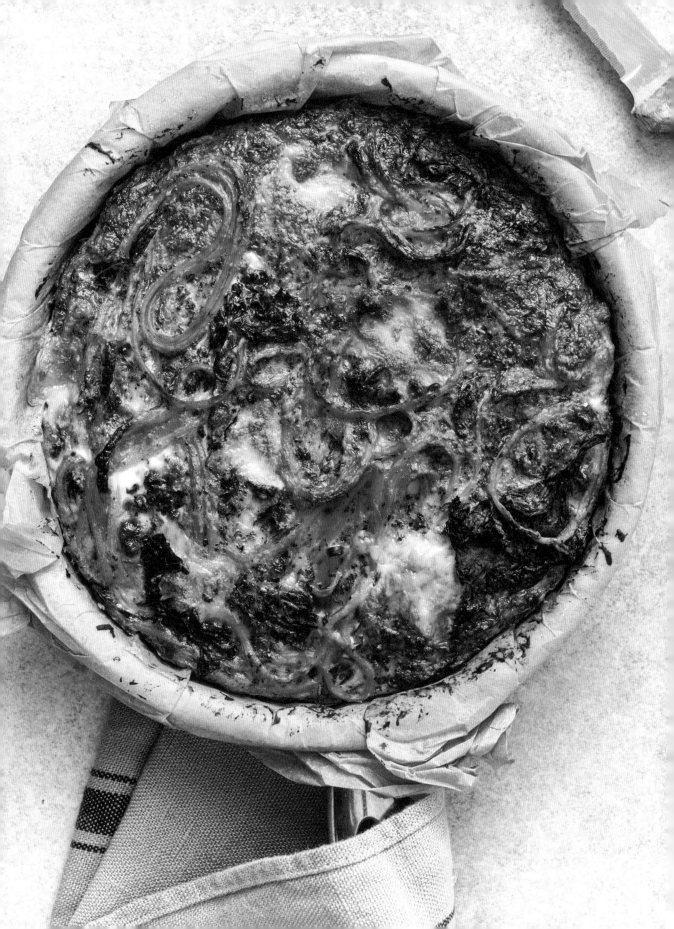

PASTA SAUCES 3 WAYS

Whenever I want a super-quick meal and find myself wavering over jars of pasta sauce, I always steel myself to walk past them and end up just making my own. Homemade pasta sauces are so much tastier, you are in control of what goes in them, and – honestly – they can be so quick to make that it's barely more effort than just opening a jar! Here are three of my top go-to pasta sauces to make at home. Each of these makes a double batch for four people, so serve up for one meal and set aside for another (or freeze if you aren't going to eat it within a few days).

VAMPIRE-LEVEL TOMATO SAUCE

**SERVES 8
(SAVE HALF THE BATCH
FOR ANOTHER MEAL)
PREP TIME: 2 MINUTES
COOK TIME: 10 MINUTES**

2 x 400g (14oz) cans of chopped
   tomatoes

8 garlic cloves

25g (1oz) basil

5 tablespoons tomato purée

1 teaspoon coarse ground salt

¼ teaspoon freshly ground
   black pepper

I love a pasta sauce with enough garlic to scare off any vampire! My favourite way of really getting that garlic flavour into sauces is to blend it up with the tomatoes. This simple pasta sauce really is just delicious and versatile: not only can you use it as a simple pasta sauce, but also as a pizza topping or a meatball sauce. This is great with a fresh chilli or two whizzed into it as well.

1   Using a stick blender or food processor, blend all the ingredients together to make a smooth sauce.

2   Simmer in a saucepan for 10 minutes. Easy!

**PER SERVING
CALORIES** 48
FAT 0.5G
SAT FAT 0G
CARBS 6.9G
SUGARS 6.3G
FIBRE 1.6G
PROTEIN 1.9G
SALT 0.73G

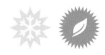

ULTRA-HERBY CREAM CHEESE SAUCE

**SERVES 8
(SAVE HALF THE BATCH
FOR ANOTHER MEAL)**
PREP TIME: 5 MINUTES
COOK TIME: 15 MINUTES

1 tablespoon dried parsley

1 teaspoon dried dill

½ teaspoon dried marjoram

½ teaspoon dried basil

½ teaspoon dried chives

¼ teaspoon dried thyme

½ teaspoon coarse ground salt

½ teaspoon garlic granules

¼ teaspoon ground black pepper

500ml (18fl oz) semi-skimmed milk

1 tbsp cornflour, stirred into a few
 tablespoons of the milk to make
 a liquid

1 vegetable stock cube or stock pot

100g (3½oz) reduced-fat cream
 cheese

30g (1oz) Parmesan-style vegetarian
 cheese, finely grated

I love the flavour of garlic and herb roulé cheese, so I've created a lighter version of it as a delicious pasta sauce. Customize this however you fancy: stir it through different pasta shapes, add chicken or bacon or fried mushrooms, or stir it through white beans and spinach.

1   Measure out all the herbs, the salt, garlic and pepper into a small bowl.

2   Put 3 tablespoons of the milk into a cup with the cornflour and stir until smooth. Pour the rest of the milk into a saucepan and place over a medium heat. Add the cornflour mixture.

3   Tip in the bowl of herbs and crumble in the stock cube (if using a stock pot, mix it with a small amount of boiling water to break it down before adding it in). Bring the milk up to a simmer, stirring.

4   Add the cream cheese and Parmesan, then simmer for 10 minutes, stirring regularly, until the sauce has thickened.

5   You can now use the sauce, keep it in the refrigerator for up to 4 days, or freeze all or half of it for another time.

PER SERVING
CALORIES 82
FAT 4G
SAT FAT 2.5G
CARBS 6.6G
SUGARS 3.5G
FIBRE 0G
PROTEIN 5G
SALT 1G

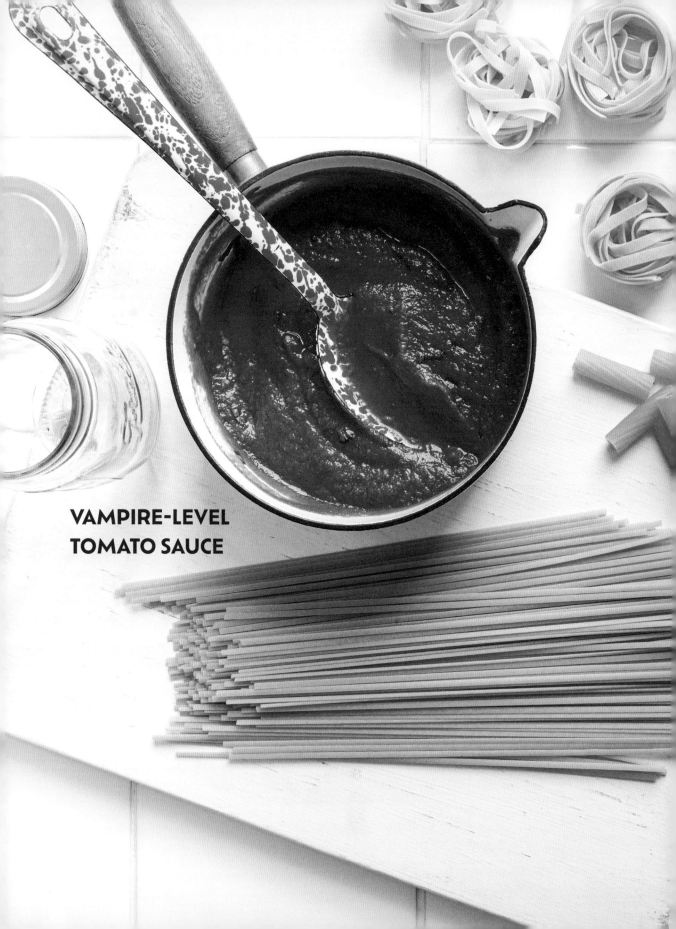

**VAMPIRE-LEVEL
TOMATO SAUCE**

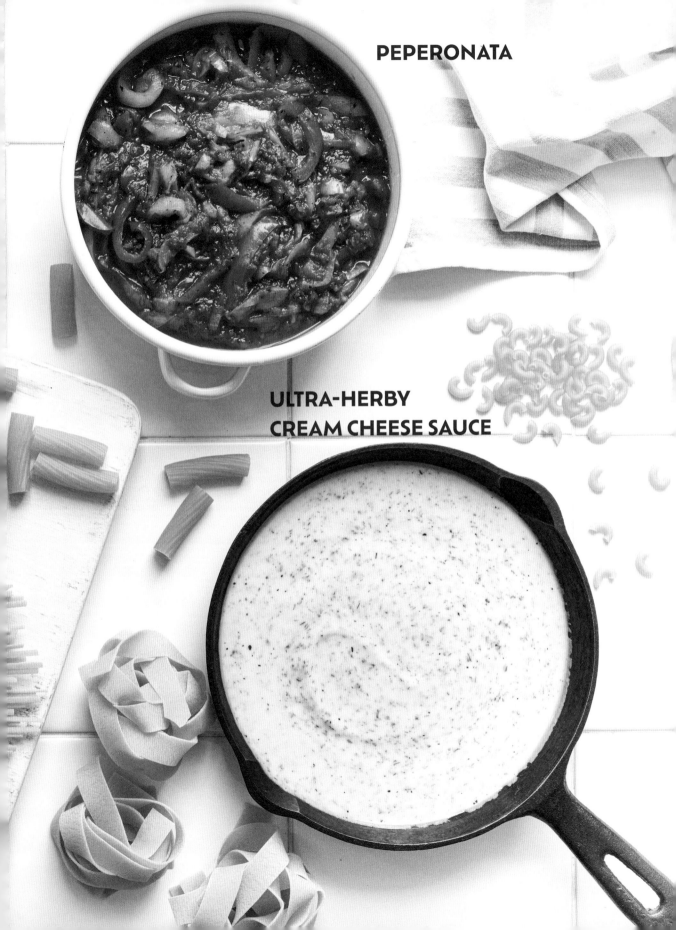

PEPERONATA

ULTRA-HERBY
CREAM CHEESE SAUCE

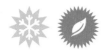

PEPERONATA

**SERVES 8
(SAVE HALF THE BATCH
FOR ANOTHER MEAL)**
PREP TIME: 10 MINUTES
COOK TIME: 50 MINUTES

1 tablespoon olive oil

1 large onion, halved and
finely sliced

6 peppers (a mix of red, orange,
yellow and green or any
combination), deseeded
and finely sliced

4 garlic cloves, crushed

400g (14oz) can of chopped
tomatoes

1 tablespoon balsamic vinegar

1 teaspoon dried basil

1 teaspoon coarse ground salt

OK, so this one isn't super-speedy, but it is very hands-off once it's cooking, and that little bit of extra cooking time brings beautiful flavours and tender consistency to this sauce. I like the peppers in this to be soft and almost falling apart, but if you prefer them to retain a little more of an al dente consistency, simply reduce the time you cook them for. As well as being a great pasta sauce, this is lovely served cold as a side dish to other meals, or is also great stuffed in a pitta bread with fried halloumi slices.

1   Heat the oil in a flameproof casserole or saucepan, which has a lid, over a medium-high heat. Stir-fry the onion for 5 minutes. Add the peppers and keep stir-frying for another 5 minutes.

2   Stir the garlic through, then add the tomatoes, balsamic vinegar, basil and salt. Place the lid on the pan and allow to simmer gently for 30 minutes, stirring occasionally.

3   Remove the lid, increase the heat to medium and simmer for 10 more minutes, allowing the sauce to thicken a little, but being careful not to allow it to stick and burn.

PER SERVING
CALORIES 83
FAT 2.2G
SAT FAT 0.3G
CARBS 11G
SUGARS 10G
FIBRE 3.7G
PROTEIN 2.2G
SALT 0.68G

Note

To make this into a meal in itself, add some canned chickpeas or cannellini beans (drained and rinsed). This is also great served over grains such as bulgur wheat or quinoa. Serving it with a fried egg on top is another great way to make it into an interesting meal.

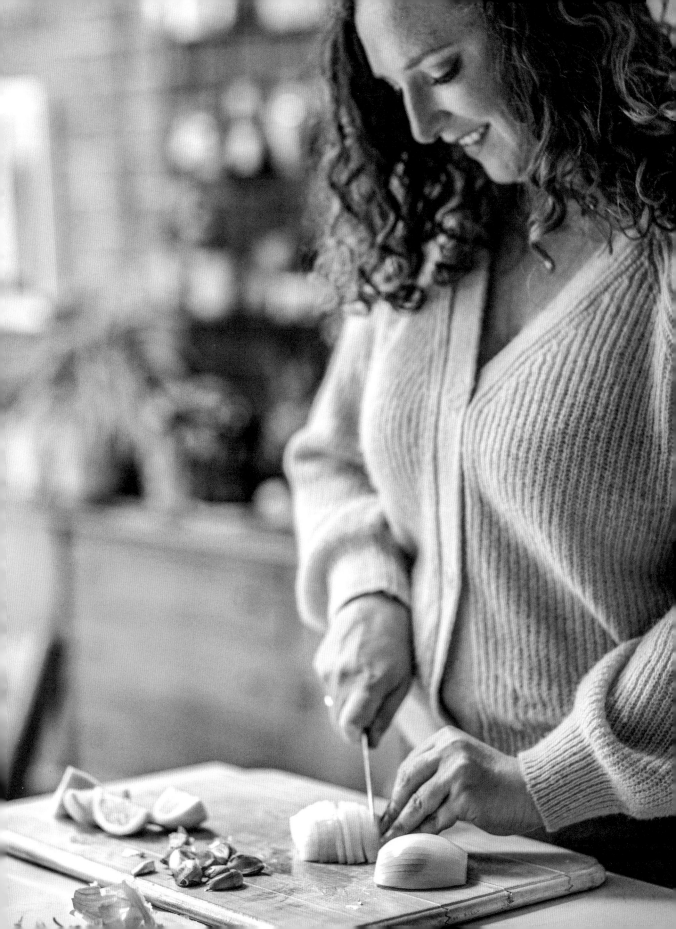

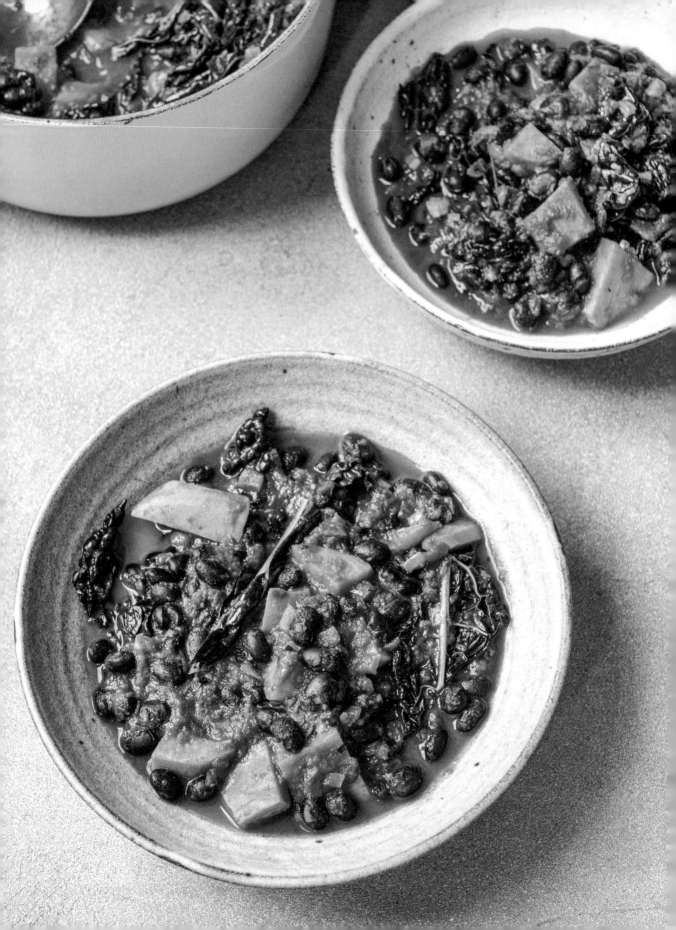

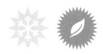

BLACK BEAN, KALE & SWEET POTATO CURRY

SERVES 2
PREP TIME: 10 MINUTES
COOK TIME: 35 MINUTES

spray oil

1 red onion, chopped

2 garlic cloves, crushed

2cm (¾ inch) piece of fresh root ginger, peeled and finely grated

½ teaspoon chilli flakes

½ teaspoon ground coriander

½ teaspoon cumin seeds

½ teaspoon ground turmeric

1 sweet potato (about 250g / 9oz), chopped

400g (14oz) can of chopped tomatoes

400g (14oz) can of black beans, drained and rinsed

300ml (½ pint) almond milk

3 large handfuls of kale, coarse stalks removed

½ teaspoon coarse ground salt

A simple curry, full of filling black beans, nutritious kale and sweet potato. This is cheap to cook and perfect for making up in a big batch so you can freeze some and reheat it for lunches. If you want to bulk it up, then add chickpeas too. If you have some of the Indian 5-spice Blend made up (see page 225), then fry a teaspoon of it in with the other ground spices here for extra depth of flavour. You can serve this with rice, or eat it on its own as bowl food.

1   Spray a sauté pan, which has a lid, with oil and place over a medium heat. Fry the onion for 5 minutes, then add the garlic and ginger and stir-fry for another minute.

2   Add all the spices, mix in, then stir in the sweet potato.

3   Tip in the chopped tomatoes, black beans, almond milk, kale and salt, cover and simmer gently for 25 minutes. Remove the lid for the last 10 minutes of cooking and give the curry a stir.

PER SERVING
CALORIES 193
FAT 2.7G
SAT FAT 0.2G
CARBS 29G
SUGARS 11G
FIBRE 8.3G
PROTEIN 8.2G
SALT 0.91G

You will find that spices are much better value if you buy them from a specialist Asian supermarket, or in the 'world foods' section of bigger supermarkets. These brands of spices come in bigger bags and are a fraction of the price of the supermarket own-brand glass jars or cardboard packets.

COURGETTE PESTO PASTA

SERVES 4
PREP TIME: 10 MINUTES
COOK TIME: 12 MINUTES

300g (10½oz) spaghetti

1 teaspoon olive oil

1 onion, finely chopped

2 medium courgettes, coarsely grated

salt and pepper

FOR THE PESTO

1 garlic clove, peeled

15g (½oz) sunflower seeds

2 teaspoons olive oil

25g (1oz) basil leaves, plus more small leaves to serve

30g (1oz) Parmesan-style vegetarian cheese, finely grated

juice of ½ lemon

large pinch of coarse ground salt

Pesto pasta is a great, cheap and simple quick meal, and here I've pepped it up with fried onion and grated courgette. Sunflower seeds make a cheap alternative to pinenuts in homemade pesto, but if you don't have time to make your own pesto, just use a ready-made variety.

1 Make the pesto by putting all the ingredients into a mini chopper and whizzing up into a paste. If it's too dry to blend properly, just add a couple of tablespoons of water.

2 Put the spaghetti on to cook according to the packet instructions.

3 Put the 1 teaspoon of olive oil in a sauté pan over a medium-low heat and start to gently fry the onion while the spaghetti cooks.

4 Stir the grated courgettes into the onion just before draining the spaghetti.

5 Drain the spaghetti and return it to the pan, add the courgettes and onion, then the freshly made pesto. Toss until the spaghetti is coated, season with salt and pepper, then serve with a few basil leaves scattered over.

PER SERVING
CALORIES 379
FAT 9G
SAT FAT 2.4G
CARBS 57G
SUGARS 6.2G
FIBRE 6.3G
PROTEIN 14G
SALT 0.52G

Note

Experiment with different pesto flavours by mixing up the herbs: you could add rosemary or sage, or even some wild garlic if it's in season. You could also try different seeds – pumpkin seeds work well – or different nuts such as cashews, walnuts and hazelnuts to add a different spin. It's a good way of using up what you have in the store cupboard.

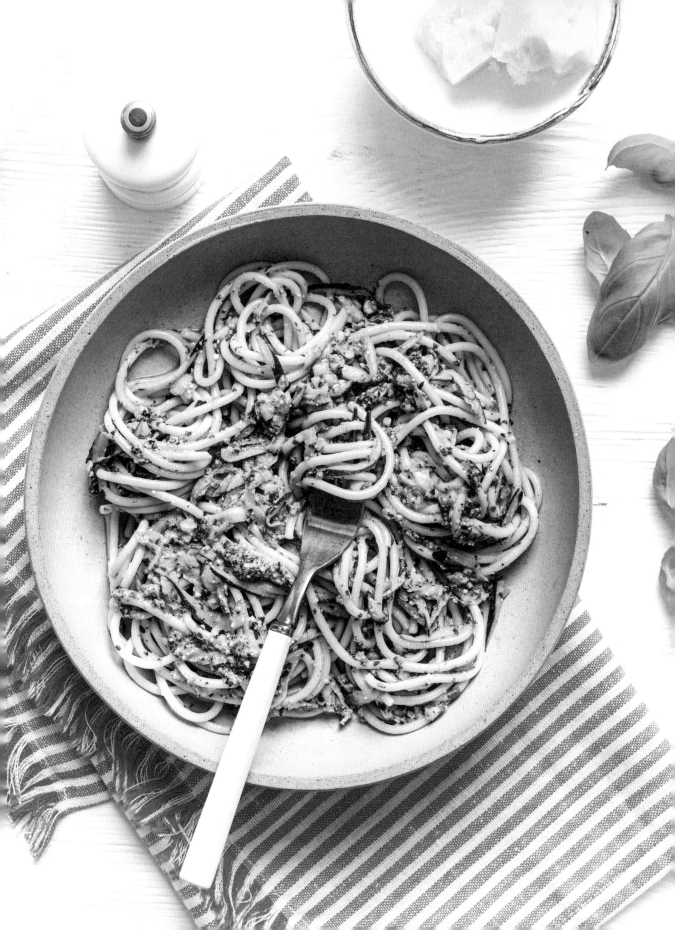

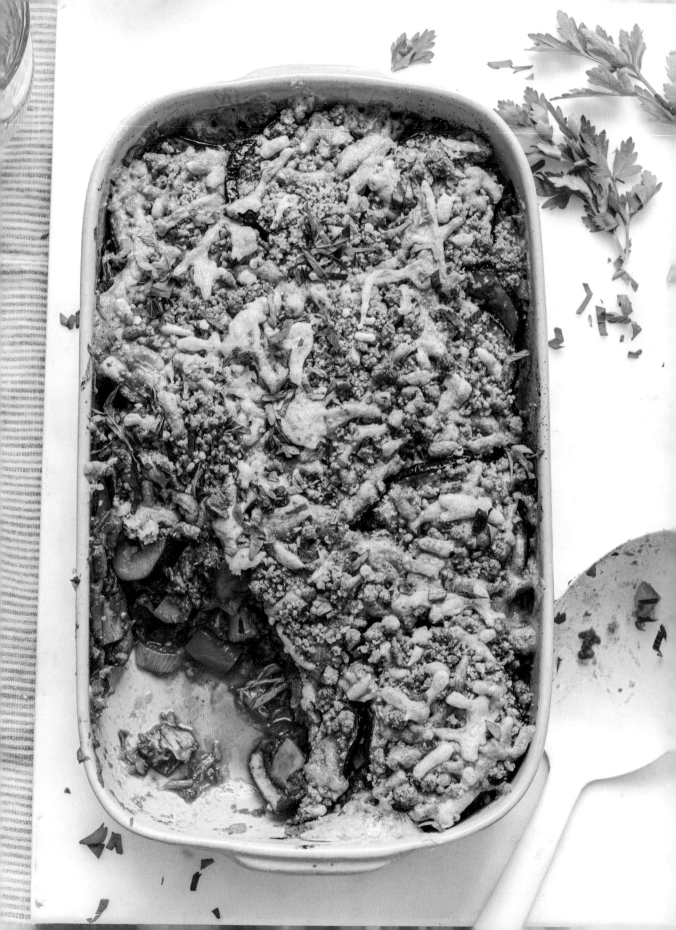

MEDITERRANEAN-STYLE TUNA & VEG CRUMBLE

spray oil, or low-calorie cooking
    spray

1 aubergine, cut into 5mm (¼ inch)
    slices

1 onion, chopped

2 garlic cloves, crushed

150g (5½oz) mushrooms, sliced

1 red pepper, deseeded and
    chopped

1 large courgette, sliced into
    half moons

2 x 145g (5¼oz) cans of tuna in
    spring water, drained

400g (14oz) can of chopped
    tomatoes

2 teaspoons Italian-style dried
    mixed herbs

1 vegetable stock cube, crumbled,
    or 1 teaspoon vegetable bouillon
    powder

1 tablespoon balsamic vinegar

chopped parsley, to garnish

salt and pepper

salad leaves, such as rocket,
    to serve

FOR THE CRUMBLE

25g (1oz) salted butter, chopped

60g (2¼oz) wholemeal flour

60g (2¼oz) mature Cheddar
    cheese, grated

This is one of those meals that is truly more than the sum of its parts. It's delicious, and hardly any extra effort to make the crumble topping. I use real butter rather than low-fat alternatives here, for two reasons: first, because you can't beat the flavour you get from just a small amount of butter; second, because this is such a healthy combination that a little butter split between four is totally worth it.

1   Pop the oven on to preheat at 200°C/180°C fan (400°F), Gas Mark 6.

2   Spray a large baking tray with oil or low-calorie cooking spray. Lay the aubergine slices out on the tray, spray them with oil or low-calorie cooking spray and put them into the oven while it's preheating and you are preparing the rest of the ingredients. Just keep half an eye on them to make sure they don't start to burn, especially if your oven is particularly quick to heat up.

3   Spray a sauté pan, which has a lid, with oil and place over a medium heat. Fry the onion, garlic, mushrooms and pepper for 8 minutes, until the onion has softened. Add the courgette and tuna, stir, then add the tomatoes, herbs, crumbled stock cube or powder, balsamic vinegar and salt and pepper. Cover and simmer gently over a low heat for 15 minutes.

4   Check on the aubergine slices, and, if they are browned and softened, remove from the oven and set aside for the moment.

5   Meanwhile, make the crumble in a bowl by rubbing the butter into the flour using your fingers until it resembles fine crumbs and there are no large lumps of butter remaining. Stir in the Cheddar.

6   Transfer the tuna and vegetable mix to a shallow ovenproof dish, arrange the softened aubergine slices over the top in an even layer, then spread the crumble mixture on top. Season with salt and pepper and place on the middle shelf of the oven to bake for 20 minutes.

7   After 20 minutes, the crumble should be golden brown and firm, but you can always leave it for a few more minutes if you think it needs a little bit more colour. Serve scattered with chopped parsley, and with some fresh salad leaves on the side.

PER SERVING

CALORIES 315
FAT 13G
SAT FAT 6.8G
CARBS 23G
SUGARS 12G
FIBRE 6.9G
PROTEIN 23G
SALT 1.9G

Note

To make a vegetarian version, leave out the tuna, add an extra red pepper and double the weight of the mushrooms.

TUNA & LEEK PASTA BAKE

SERVES 4
PREP TIME: 8 MINUTES
COOK TIME: 30 MINUTES

300g penne pasta

spray oil

3 spring onions, sliced, plus more
    to serve

2 large leeks, trimmed, cleaned and
    sliced

1 chicken stock pot or stock cube

1 teaspoon dried oregano

1 teaspoon mustard powder

100g (3½oz) reduced-fat cream
    cheese

2 x 145g (5¼oz) cans tuna in spring
    water, drained

120g (4½oz) mature Cheddar
    cheese, grated

1 head of broccoli, cut into florets

salt and pepper

snipped chives or chopped parsley
    leaves, to serve

This meal is so quick and easy to throw together. It's great comfort food, full of flavour and goodness. Sometimes I use wholemeal pasta – or even a mix of white and wholemeal – and you can use whatever pasta shapes you fancy.

1 Preheat the oven to 220°C/200°C fan (425°F), Gas Mark 7.

2 Put the pasta on to boil in a large pan of water and cook according to the packet instructions. You need to make sure you have plenty of water in the pan, as you will use some of the pasta water to make up the sauce.

3 Spray a sauté pan or a flameproof shallow casserole dish with oil and place over a medium-low heat. Fry the spring onions and leeks gently while the pasta cooks.

4 When the pasta is nearly cooked, make up the chicken stock pot in a jug using a couple of ladles of the pasta water (about 200ml/7fl oz). Drain the pasta.

5 Pour the hot chicken stock into the leeks, then stir in the oregano and mustard powder. Add the pasta to the pan, then the cream cheese, stirring this into the hot pasta and allowing it to melt. Add the tuna and half the grated cheese, season with salt and pepper and mix everything together.

6 Transfer into an ovenproof dish (if your current pan or dish is not ovenproof) and scatter the broccoli over the top. Cover with the remaining grated cheese and spray with a little spray oil.

7 Bake for 15 minutes, until the cheese on top is melted and golden. Serve scattered with the spring onions, chives or parsley.

PER SERVING
CALORIES 548
FAT 16G
SAT FAT 8.9G
CARBS 60G
SUGARS 6.9G
FIBRE 7.1G
PROTEIN 38G
SALT 2.1G

Note

Want to get extra fibre and filling-power in this pasta bake? You could add a can of white beans such as butter beans, cannellini or haricot. Simply stir the beans into the cheese sauce before it goes in the oven. A few large handfuls of baby spinach leaves stirred into the sauce also works well.

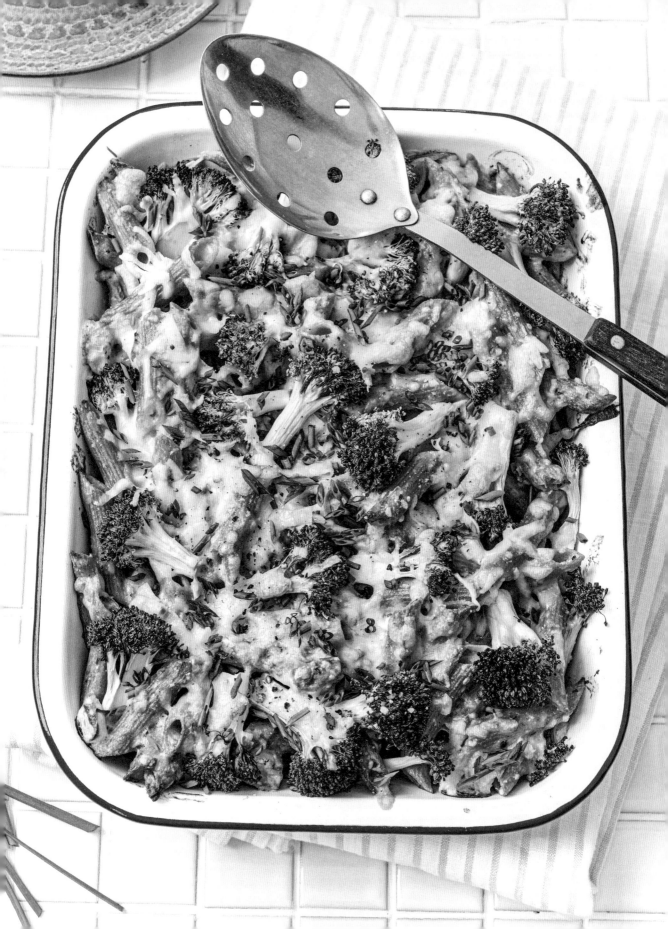

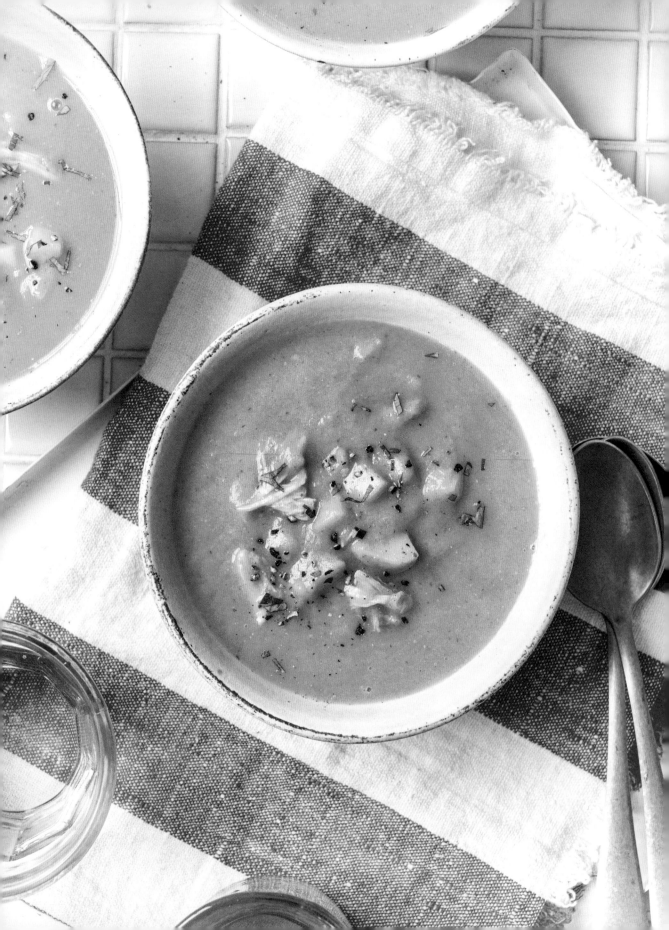

SOUL-FOOD SWEET POTATO & CHICKEN SOUP

SERVES 4
PREP TIME: 10 MINUTES
COOK TIME: 45 MINUTES

spray oil

2 skinless chicken thigh fillets

1 onion, chopped

1 leek, trimmed, cleaned and sliced

1–2 large sweet potatoes (total weight about 500g / 1lb 2oz), chopped

1 large carrot, sliced

1 garlic clove, crushed

1 litre (1¾ pints) hot chicken stock (see note below)

about 15g (½oz) parsley stalks and leaves, chopped

400g (14oz) potatoes, peeled and finely chopped (into about 5mm / ¼ inch cubes)

salt and pepper

You only need a small amount of chicken to make this soothing and vitamin-packed soup. The sweet potato gives it rich flavour and a thick, comforting consistency, while the chicken and regular potato lend it texture as well as extra filling power. This is my kids' favourite soup... and all the vegetables are blended, so it's great for picky eaters! With this soup I tend to throw the ingredients in as I chop them, rather than pre-preparing all the veg.

1   Start by spraying a deep, flameproof casserole with oil. Place over a medium heat and start to fry the chicken. Add the onion, then the leek and let those fry gently for 5–10 minutes while you chop the sweet potatoes and carrot.

2   Add the garlic to the casserole with the sweet potatoes and carrot, then pour in the chicken stock. Add the parsley, bring to the boil, then reduce the heat to a simmer and leave to simmer for 20 minutes.

3   Remove the chicken from the pot and set aside for a moment, while you use a stick blender to whizz up the soup to a smooth consistency.

4   Thinly slice the cooked chicken, chop it into small pieces, then pop it back into the soup along with the regular potatoes. Leave to simmer for another 15 minutes until the regular potato pieces are tender.

5   Season to taste with salt and pepper: the right level of salt will really affect the flavour of this, so if it's a little bland you might just need to add a tad more. It is now ready to serve.

PER SERVING
CALORIES 332
FAT 2.8G
SAT FAT 0.8G
CARBS 49G
SUGARS 13G
FIBRE 7.7G
PROTEIN 23G
SALT 1.9G

Note

I often make this if we have had roast chicken and there's a little meat left over, but not enough for a full meal. I very finely chop whatever chicken we have and throw it in after I've made and blended the soup. I just miss out cooking the chicken thighs in step 1. This is extra-delicious with homemade chicken stock, if you have some.

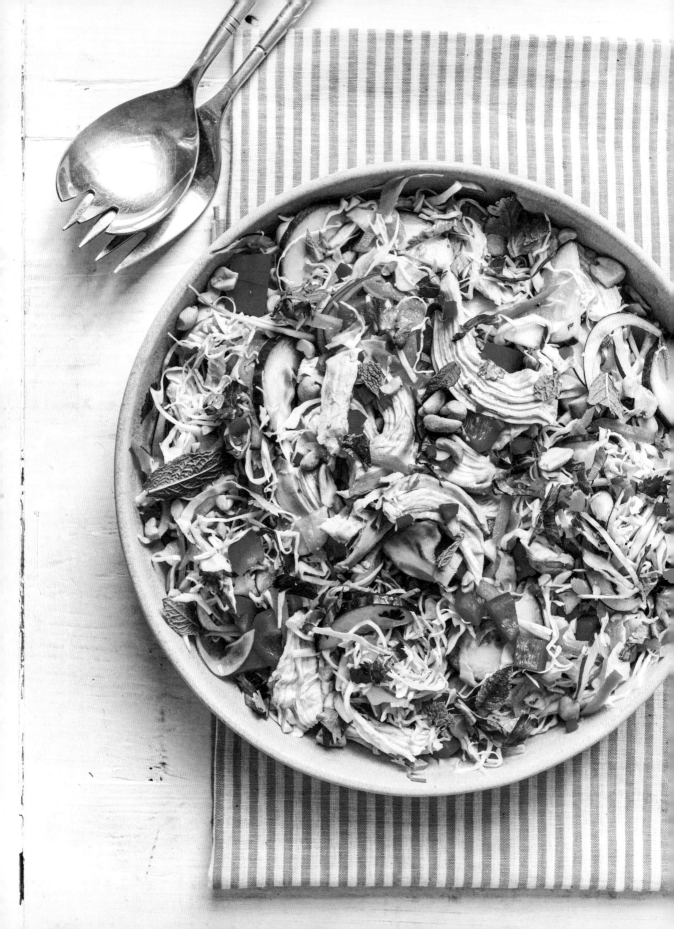

SERVES 4
PREP TIME: 15 MINUTES
COOK TIME: 12 MINUTES

2 skinless chicken breasts

2 tablespoons dark soy sauce

1 pointed spring cabbage,
    thinly sliced

2 large carrots, grated

½ red onion, thinly sliced

1 red pepper, deseeded and
    finely chopped

½ cucumber, halved lengthways
    and thinly sliced into half moons

1 red chilli, deseeded and
    finely chopped

large handful of mint leaves,
    finely shredded

large handful of coriander leaves
    and stems, finely chopped

50g (1¾oz) unsalted peanuts,
    lightly crushed

salt and pepper

FOR THE DRESSING

juice of 1 lime

2 tablespoons rice vinegar

2 tablespoons fish sauce

1 tablespoon sweet chilli sauce

1 garlic clove, crushed

CRUNCHY VIETNAMESE-STYLE CHICKEN SALAD

This is a really satisfying salad, with plenty of crunch and texture complemented by a punchy dressing. A little bit of meat goes a long way here, so the recipe is a great way to use up leftover roast chicken, if you have it. I tend to prepare the veg while the chicken is poaching, to make the most efficient use of my time.

1   Place the chicken breasts in a saucepan and just cover with water. Add the dark soy sauce, bring to the boil, then simmer for 12 minutes while you prepare the rest of the dish.

2   Make the dressing by mixing all the ingredients in a small bowl.

3   In a large serving bowl, use your hands or salad servers to toss together the cabbage, carrots, red onion, red pepper, cucumber, chilli and herbs.

4   When the chicken is ready, cut the breasts in half to check they are cooked all the way through, then slice them up as thinly as you can. Add the chicken to the salad bowl, season with salt and pepper, pour over the dressing, then toss the sliced chicken and dressing through the salad.

5   Top with the peanuts and serve.

PER SERVING

CALORIES 251

FAT 8.3G

SAT FAT 1.4G

CARBS 15G

SUGARS 14G

FIBRE 5.5G

PROTEIN 27G

SALT 2.9G

 Note

> You can buy pre-cooked chicken to add to this if you want a quicker option, and you could add cooked rice noodles for more filling power.

> For a vegetarian version, replace the chicken with fried tofu. Drain and pat dry 250g (9oz) firm tofu with kitchen paper, then cut into 1cm (½ inch) cubes. Heat 1 tablespoon oil in a frying pan and stir-fry the tofu cubes for 10 minutes until golden. Toss these through the salad instead of the chicken and replace the fish sauce with a vegetarian/vegan alternative.

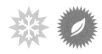

PARMIGIANA DI MELANZANE

SERVES 4
PREP TIME: 10 MINUTES
COOK TIME: 55 MINUTES

spray oil, or low-calorie cooking
    spray

3 large aubergines, sliced
    lengthways as thinly as you can

1 large onion, chopped

4 garlic cloves, crushed

500ml (18fl oz) tomato passata

1 teaspoon Italian seasoning

200g (7oz) mozzarella cheese,
    torn into small pieces

60g (2¼oz) Parmesan-style
    vegetarian cheese, finely grated

salt and pepper

This baked aubergine, tomato, mozzarella and Parmesan dish is one of my favourite Italian meals. It's a dish where all the flavours and textures just blend perfectly into something really special. Traditionally the aubergine is salted, coated in flour, then fried in plenty of olive oil. To simplify this for us home cooks, I prefer to bake the aubergine slices. You can still achieve a tender texture this way and it's also hands-off, so you can make a quick tomato sauce while the aubergine is cooking. Serve this with a simple side of rocket and balsamic glaze.

1   Preheat the oven to 220°C/200°C fan (425°F), Gas Mark 7.

2   Line 2 baking trays with nonstick baking paper and spray lightly with spray oil or low-calorie cooking spray. Lie the aubergine slices over the baking trays in a single layer, spray them with spray oil or low-calorie cooking spray (spray is great for this recipe as it gives good all-over coverage), then season with salt and pepper. Place in the oven and bake for 20 minutes while you make the tomato sauce.

3   Fry the onion in spray oil or low-calorie cooking spray for 10 minutes, until it is softened and golden brown. Stir in the crushed garlic and cook with the onion for the last minute. Pour in the passata, add the Italian seasoning, then season to taste with salt and pepper. Simmer the tomato sauce while the aubergine bakes, allowing it to reduce slightly and stirring every now and again.

4   In an ovenproof baking dish (I use my lasagne dish for this), layer up the Parmigiana, starting with one-third of the tomato sauce, then a layer of one-third of the aubergine slices, then one-third of the mozzarella pieces and one-third of the Parmesan. Repeat this pattern to use up all the ingredients, finishing with a layer of cheese.

5   Cover with foil and bake in the oven for 20 minutes.

6   Remove the foil and cook for another 10–15 minutes uncovered, until you have a bubbling, golden-brown cheesy crust on top.

PER SERVING
CALORIES 329
FAT 16G
SAT FAT 10G
CARBS 19G
SUGARS 16G
FIBRE 8.3G
PROTEIN 20G
SALT 1.1G

> You can use a mix of courgette and aubergine for this dish if you prefer (bake the courgette in the same way as the aubergine).

> Use a Bolognese sauce instead of the tomato sauce, if you want to add some meat (for my homemade Ultimate Bolognese sauce, see page 180).

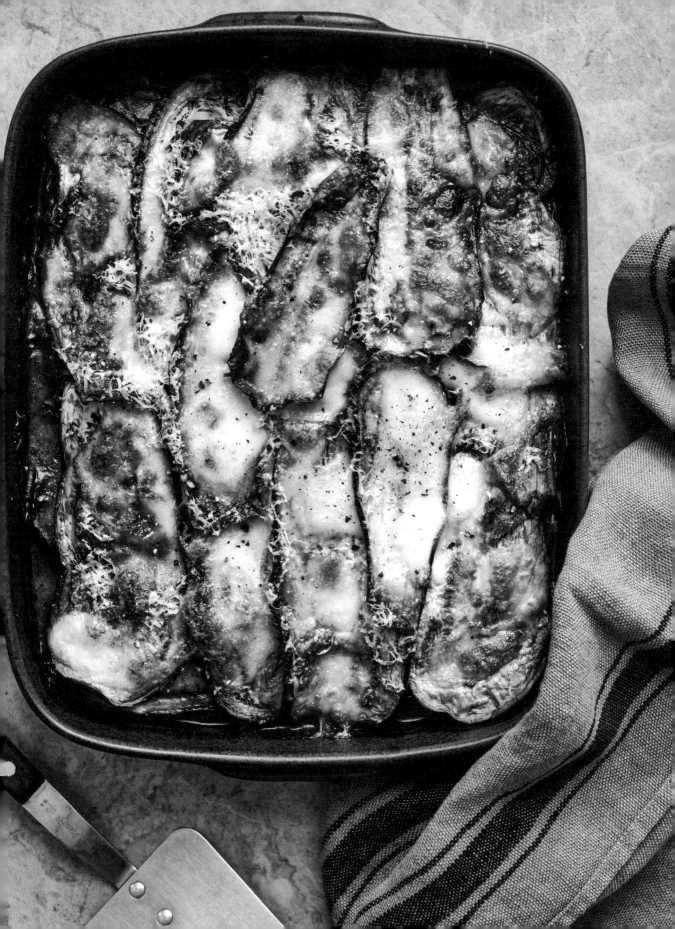

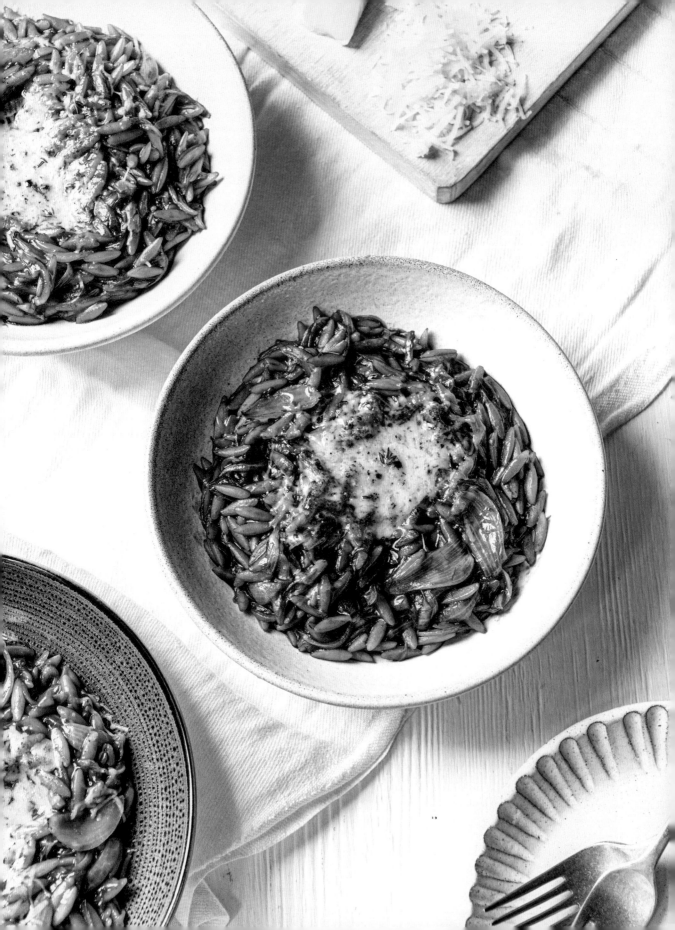

FRENCH ONION ORZOTTO

SERVES 4
PREP TIME: 10 MINUTES
COOK TIME: 45 MINUTES

1 tablespoon butter

1 teaspoon olive oil

4 large onions, peeled and very finely sliced

2 garlic cloves, crushed

1 teaspoon coarse ground salt

1 litre (1¾ pints) hot beef stock

300g (10½oz) orzo

1 tablespoon Worcestershire sauce, plus more to serve

1 teaspoon dried thyme

120g (4¼oz) Gruyère cheese, grated

freshly ground black pepper

French onion soup is so delicious that I decided to use the key flavours of rich, golden onions and melty Gruyère cheese to make it into a more substantial meal with orzo. This is so simple and – as a bonus – also low cost! You do need a small amount of butter and oil just to get the onions perfectly melting and caramelized, but it's totally worth it. For a vegetable side dish, asparagus or crunchy green beans go well. If you are feeling indulgent, French bread is a great treat alongside this meal.

1   Melt the butter with the oil in a medium saucepan. Add the onions and toss them around to coat them in the butter and oil, then fry them gently, stirring often, for 25 minutes. They should be soft and caramel-coloured.

2   Stir in the garlic and salt, then pour in the beef stock and add the orzo, Worcestershire sauce, thyme and a few grinds of pepper.

3   Stir well and allow to simmer gently for 15 minutes, stirring every now and again to make sure that the orzo isn't sticking to the bottom of the pan. (If you find that the orzo is becoming too dry – the size and shape of your pan can affect this – then just pour in a little hot water.)

4   After 15 minutes, try a bit of orzo to check it is cooked through. Give it a few more minutes of simmering if it has too much bite. Stir through half the Gruyère cheese to melt it, while you preheat the grill to high.

5   Divide between 4 flameproof bowls, sprinkle the rest of the Gruyère over the top, drizzle over a little Worcestershire sauce, then pop the bowls under a hot grill for a few minutes to get the cheese on top golden brown and bubbling. Serve immediately.

PER SERVING
CALORIES 557
FAT 16G
SAT FAT 8.6G
CARBS 7.4G
SUGARS 19G
FIBRE 8.8G
PROTEIN 24G
SALT 3.3G

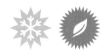

SIMPLE RED LENTIL DAL

SERVES 4
PREP TIME: 10 MINUTES
COOK TIME: 40 MINUTES

spray oil

1 large onion, finely chopped

3 large garlic cloves, crushed

3cm (1¼ inch) piece of fresh root ginger, peeled and finely grated

1 green chilli, deseeded and finely chopped

1 teaspoon cumin seeds

½ teaspoon mustard seeds

1 teaspoon ground turmeric

400g (14oz) can of chopped tomatoes

160g (5¾oz) dried red lentils

450ml (16fl oz) hot vegetable stock

½ teaspoon coarse ground salt

¼ teaspoon freshly ground black pepper

juice of 1 lemon

coriander leaves, to serve (optional)

It's always good to have a simple dal recipe on hand, because it's such a cheap, satisfying, versatile, nutritious and delicious dish. For a filling meal, you can serve this with rice, naan bread or pitta bread, but it's delicious just on its own as well. It's also worth knocking up a big batch and keeping some portions in the freezer, then, when you are cooking up a different curry, you can simply defrost them to use as a side dish.

1   Spray the oil into a large saucepan and place over a medium heat. Cook the onion for 5 minutes, until it has softened. Add the garlic, ginger, chilli, cumin seeds, mustard seeds and turmeric and cook for 1 minute. Add the chopped tomatoes and stir thoroughly into the onion and spices.

2   Tip in the red lentils and vegetable stock, bring to a simmer and season with the salt and pepper.

3   Cover and simmer for 30 minutes, stirring every now and again, until the lentils are soft and cooked through, with no bite to them.

4   Stir through the lemon juice and serve, scattered with coriander, if you like.

PER SERVING
CALORIES 212
FAT 1.8G
SAT FAT 0.4G
CARBS 32G
SUGARS 11G
FIBRE 5.4G
PROTEIN 12G
SALT 0.82G

Note

To make this a little more indulgent and creamier, replace the vegetable stock with light coconut milk.

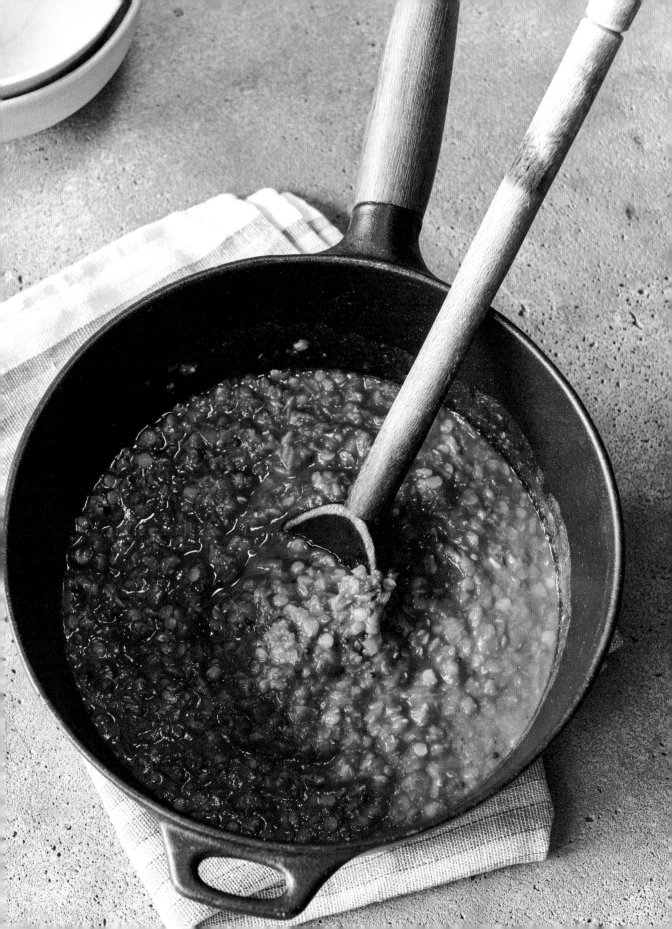

- ✓ ASAM PEDAS (SOUR-SPICY MALAYSIAN FISH CURRY)
- ✓ KING PRAWN BIRYANI
- ✓ TAMARIND PRAWN CURRY
- ✓ RANCHERO MAC 'N' CHEESE
- ✓ RICH, TOMATOEY CHICKEN AND AUBERGINE CURRY
- ✓ STIR-FRIED CHAR SUI PORK WITH UDON NOODLES
- ✓ SWEET AND SOUR PORK
- ✓ SPICED LAMB AND AUBERGINE RICE WITH MINTY YOGURT
- ✓ BEEF AND BLACK BEAN BURGERS WITH HOT CORN SALSA
- ✓ CHILLI-PEANUT BEEF AND NOODLES
- ✓ CHICKEN AND SWEET POTATO VINDALOO

5

Feasting Friday

ASAM PEDAS (SOUR-SPICY MALAYSIAN FISH CURRY)

SERVES 4
PREP TIME: 15 MINUTES
COOK TIME: 25 MINUTES

1 onion, quartered

2 garlic cloves, peeled

2cm (¾ inch) piece of fresh root ginger, peeled and roughly chopped

1 red chilli, deseeded and roughly chopped

15g (½oz) bunch of coriander, stems finely chopped, leaves set aside

1 teaspoon ground coriander

1 teaspoon ground cumin

½ teaspoon ground turmeric

spray oil

1 teaspoon black mustard seeds (or brown if you can't find black)

2 salad tomatoes, quartered

200ml (7fl oz) water

2 tablespoons tamarind paste

175g (6oz) okra, trimmed

250g (9oz) jasmine rice

½ teaspoon coarse ground salt

¼ teaspoon freshly ground black pepper

4 fresh white fish fillets, such as hake, cod or haddock

This is my take on a very special curry which is grounded in the sourness of tamarind and spiciness of chilli. In the UK, it's not easy to get hold of some of the authentic spices which are integral to the amazing flavours in Malaysian cuisine. However, tamarind paste is widely available, and by using other ingredients that we *can* find in our shops, it's still possible to create a delicious sour and spicy Malaysian-inspired fish curry.

1   In a mini chopper, blend together the onion, garlic, ginger, chilli, coriander stems, ground coriander, cumin and turmeric to make a paste.

2   Spray a sauté pan, which has a lid, with oil and set over a medium-high heat. Add the mustard seeds, cook them for about 1 minute until they just start sizzling, then add the curry paste, give it a good stir and let it fry gently for about 4 minutes.

3   Meanwhile, add the tomato quarters to the mini chopper and whizz them up into a purée. Stir the tomatoes into the curry paste, then add the measured water, bring to a simmer, then stir in the tamarind paste.

4   Add the okra to the sauce, place the lid on the pan and leave to simmer for 10 minutes.

5   Cook the jasmine rice according to the packet instructions.

6   After the sauce has simmered for 10 minutes, stir in the salt and pepper, lay the fish fillets on top, place the lid back on and simmer for another 5–8 minutes until the fish is cooked through. (To test whether your fish is done, you can insert a fork at an angle at the thickest point and give it a little twist: when it is cooked it will flake easily and will have lost its translucent/raw appearance.)

7   Divide the cooked jasmine rice between 4 plates and top each portion with a fish fillet, the sauce and okra. Scatter the coriander leaves over to serve.

PER SERVING
CALORIES 395
FAT 2.4G
SAT FAT 0.5G
CARBS 59G
SUGARS 7.4G
FIBRE 4.7G
PROTEIN 32G
SALT 1.5G

Note

If you can't get hold of okra, you could substitute green beans, courgette or broccoli. If using any of these alternatives, give them 5 minutes less cooking time than the okra (so add them after the sauce has been simmering for 5 minutes.)

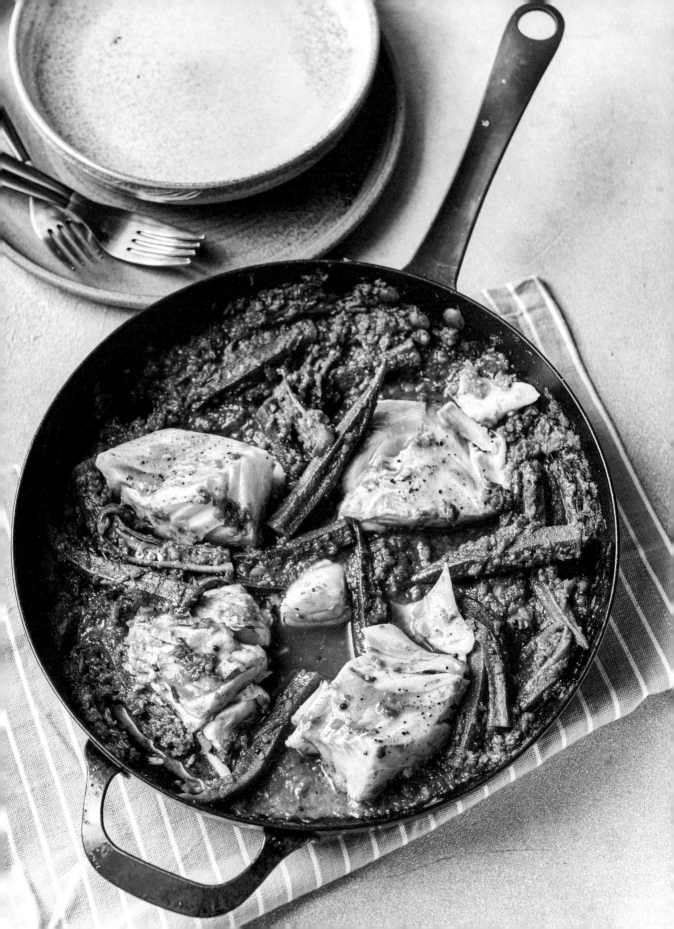

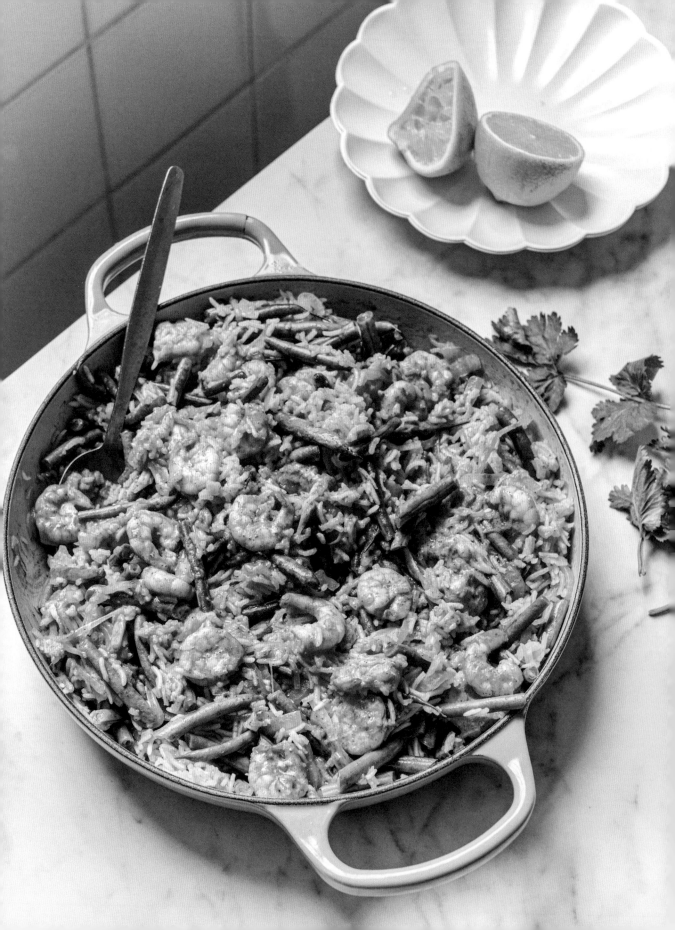

KING PRAWN BIRIYANI

SERVES 4
PREP TIME: 10 MINUTES
COOK TIME: 30 MINUTES

300g (10½oz) cooked and peeled king prawns

1 teaspoon chilli powder (mild or hot, to taste)

½ teaspoon coarse ground salt

½ teaspoon ground turmeric

3 tablespoons fat-free Greek yogurt

1 tablespoon vegetable oil or olive oil

2 large onions, finely sliced

2.5cm (1 inch) piece of fresh root ginger, peeled and finely grated

1 garlic clove, crushed

1 tablespoon tomato purée

300g (10½oz) basmati rice, rinsed under cold water until the water runs clear

850ml (1½ pints) hot chicken stock

300g (10½oz) fine green beans, topped and tailed and cut into 2cm pieces

juice of ½ lemon

handful of coriander leaves, chopped

Tender king prawns in fragrant rice make this easy, one-pot biriyani a great family-friendly Friday feast!

1 In a bowl, mix the prawns, chilli powder, salt, turmeric and yogurt. Set aside.

2 Heat the vegetable oil or olive oil, in a pan that has a lid over a medium-low heat. Fry the sliced onions in the oil for 10 minutes, until soft and golden. Stir in the ginger and garlic, fry for 1 minute, then stir in the tomato purée and fry for another minute.

3 Stir the rice into the pan, then pour in the chicken stock. Bring to a simmer, then cover, reduce the heat and simmer for 10 minutes, so that the rice is simmering very gently. Give the rice a stir halfway through.

4 Now stir the green beans through the rice, then the prawns and their marinade. Cover with the lid again and simmer gently for 5 more minutes.

5 Remove the lid and stir in the lemon juice. The rice should be cooked through and tender. Serve scattered with coriander.

PER SERVING
CALORIES 468
FAT 5.1G
SAT FAT 1G
CARBS 72G
SUGARS 11G
FIBRE 7.1G
PROTEIN 29G
SALT 2.9G

TAMARIND PRAWN CURRY

SERVES 4
PREP TIME: 10 MINUTES
COOK TIME: 25 MINUTES

1 teaspoon vegetable oil

1 large onion, finely sliced

240g (8½oz) jasmine rice

250g (9oz) cherry tomatoes

3 garlic cloves, crushed

3cm (1¼ inch) piece of fresh root
  ginger, peeled and finely grated

2 birdseye chillies, deseeded and
  finely chopped

1 teaspoon nigella seeds

1 teaspoon cumin seeds

1 teaspoon ground turmeric

360g (12½oz) raw king prawns

large handful of coriander, stalks
  and leaves chopped separately

200g (7oz) tomato passata

1 tablespoon tamarind paste

1 lime, cut into wedges, to serve
  (optional)

A tangy and spicy curry with juicy prawns, served over steaming jasmine rice.

1   Heat the oil in a sauté pan over a medium-high heat, then fry the onion for 6 minutes. Meanwhile, put the jasmine rice on to cook (see note below).

2   Add the cherry tomatoes to the onions and fry for another 3 minutes. Add the garlic, ginger and chillies and stir-fry for 1 minute. Add the nigella seeds, cumin seeds and turmeric and stir-fry for another 30 seconds.

3   Now tip in the prawns and coriander stalks and stir-fry for about 3 minutes, until the prawns turn pink, then stir in the passata and tamarind. Gently simmer for 10 minutes.

4   While the curry is simmering, drain the jasmine rice, put it back in the pan, cover and leave it to steam until the curry is ready.

5   Fluff up the rice with a fork, divide between 4 plates, then serve the curry. Scatter with the coriander leaves and serve with the lime wedges if liked.

PER SERVING
CALORIES 373
FAT 3.2G
SAT FAT 0.4G
CARBS 60G
SUGARS 10G
FIBRE 4G
PROTEIN 22G
SALT 1.7G

Note

To cook perfect jasmine rice, bring a large saucepan of water to the boil. Pour in the jasmine rice (allow 60g / 2¼oz rice per person). Reduce the heat to low, cover the pan and cook for 12 minutes. Drain the rice, put it back into the pan with the lid on, then leave it to steam for another 3 minutes. Fluff it through with a fork before serving.

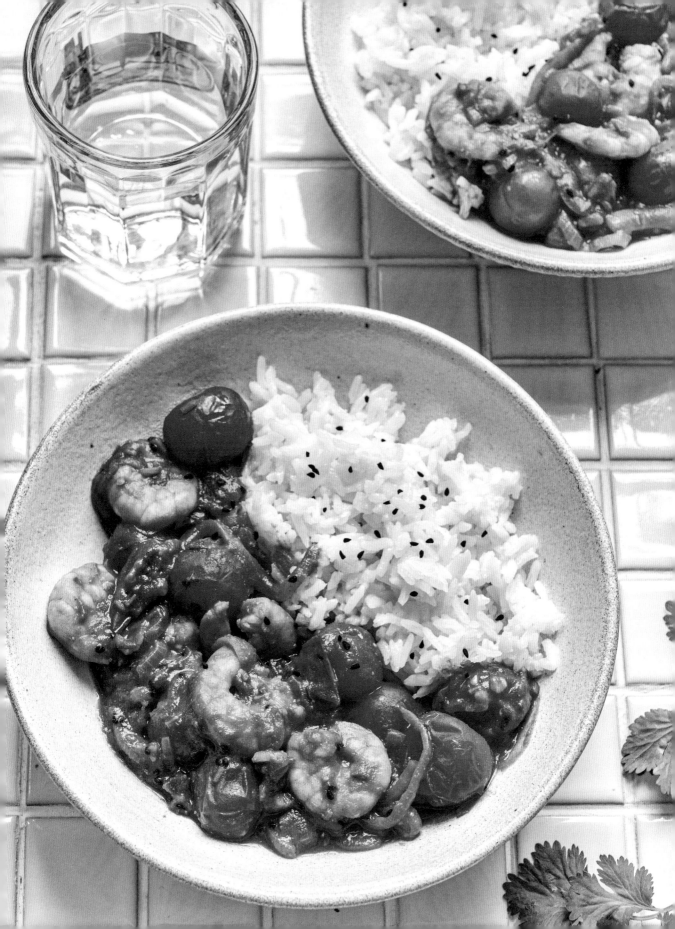

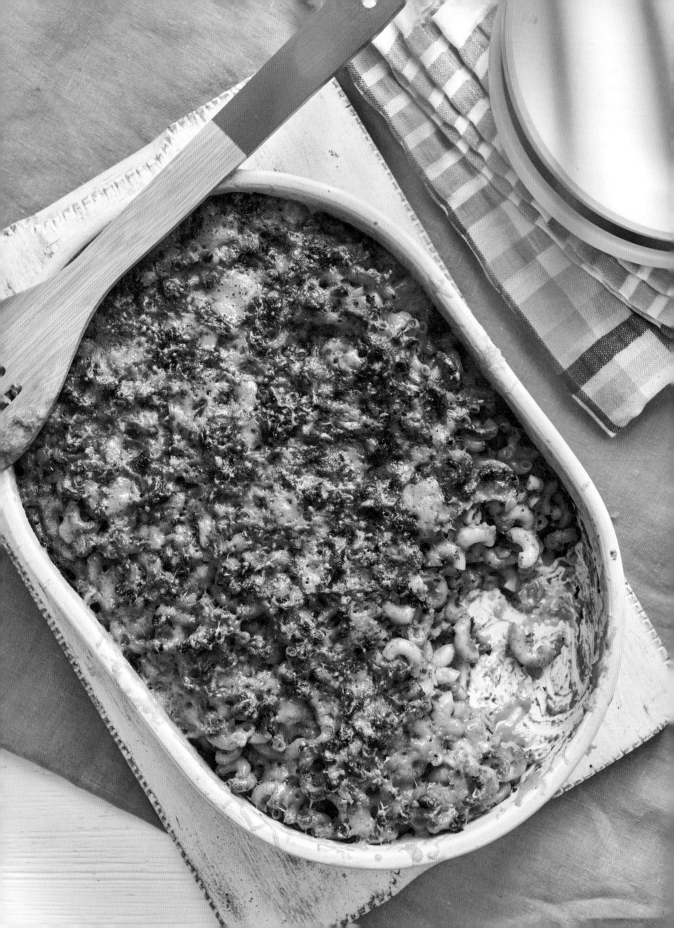

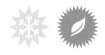

RANCHERO MAC 'N' CHEESE

SERVES 4
PREP TIME: 5 MINUTES
COOK TIME: 40 MINUTES

spray oil

1 red onion, chopped

400g (14oz) can of chopped
tomatoes

1 tablespoon chopped pickled
jalapeños

250ml (9fl oz) hot vegetable or
chicken stock

small handful of coriander leaves
and stems, roughly chopped

1 teaspoon chipotle chilli paste
(or see recipe introduction)

1 teaspoon dried oregano

1 teaspoon ground cumin

½ teaspoon garlic granules

juice of 1 lime

300g (10½oz) macaroni

3 tablespoons reduced-fat cream
cheese

120g (4¼oz) red Leicester (or other
vegetarian cheese), grated

salt and pepper

Ranchero sauce is a Tex-Mex tomato and chilli sauce, which makes
an incredible flavourful base for a mac 'n' cheese with a twist. Many
supermarkets sell chipotle chilli paste, which has a distinctive smoky
flavour, though ancho chilli paste would be a good substitute if that's
easier for you to find. If you want to add a side dish, then my Hot Corn
Salsa (see page 131) works well with this.

1   Start by making the ranchero sauce. Spray a frying pan with oil and place
    it over a medium-low heat. Fry the onion for 10 minutes to soften and
    brown it. Add the tomatoes, jalapeños, stock, coriander, chipotle paste,
    oregano, cumin, garlic granules and lime juice, season with salt and
    pepper and simmer for 20 minutes, stirring every now and again.

2   Meanwhile, cook the macaroni according to the packet instructions,
    then drain (reserving a little of the cooking water), put back into the pan
    and set aside until the sauce is ready.

3   Transfer the ranchero sauce to a blender or food processor and whizz it
    until it's smooth. Preheat the grill to high.

4   Turn the heat on low under the macaroni pan, pour in the sauce, add the
    cream cheese and stir everything together until the cream cheese has
    melted. Add a little of the reserved pasta cooking water if you need
    some liquid to loosen it up a little. Add half the red Leicester and stir
    it through.

5   Transfer the coated pasta to an ovenproof dish and use the remaining
    red Leicester cheese to cover the top. Place the dish under the hot grill
    and grill for 7–8 minutes, until the cheese on top is melted and bubbling.

PER SERVING

CALORIES 526
FAT 17G
SAT FAT 8.7G
CARBS 67G
SUGARS 15G
FIBRE 7.2G
PROTEIN 21G
SALT 2.1G

Note

If you want to add some extra veggies to this, you could try thinly sliced roasted pepper or a can of
sweetcorn, tipping them in when you stir the sauce into the pasta. You could also bulk the dish up
by adding a drained can of pinto beans or black beans at this stage.

RICH, TOMATOEY CHICKEN & AUBERGINE CURRY

SERVES 4
PREP TIME: 15 MINUTES
COOK TIME: 45 MINUTES

1 aubergine, cut into chunks

2 large red onions, finely chopped

3 chicken breasts (total weight about 450g / 1lb), cut into chunks

3 garlic cloves, crushed

3cm (1¼ inch) piece of fresh root ginger, peeled and finely grated

2 teaspoons cumin seeds

3 tablespoons tomato purée

400g (14oz) can of chopped tomatoes

2 tablespoons honey

1 teaspoon chilli flakes

1 tablespoon tamarind paste

1 teaspoon coarse ground salt

¼ tsp freshly ground black pepper

300ml (½ pint) hot water

handful of coriander leaves, to serve (optional)

A tasty, saucy curry with sweet and sour flavours, this is lovely served simply with flatbread or pitta, or white or brown rice.

1 Spray a sauté pan with oil, place over a medium-high heat and fry the aubergine chunks and red onion for 8 minutes.

2 Add the chicken and stir-fry for another 3 minutes.

3 Stir in the garlic, ginger and cumin seeds, fry for 1 minute, then add the tomato purée and stir-fry everything for 2 more minutes. Add the chopped tomatoes to the pan, then stir in the honey, chilli, tamarind paste, salt and pepper.

4 Stir the measured water into the pan, bring to the boil, then reduce the heat to a simmer. Leave to simmer for 30 minutes, stirring occasionally. Serve scattered with coriander leaves if liked.

PER SERVING
CALORIES 249
FAT 2.3G
SAT FAT 0.5G
CARBS 22G
SUGARS 19G
FIBRE 4G
PROTEIN 31G
SALT 1.8G

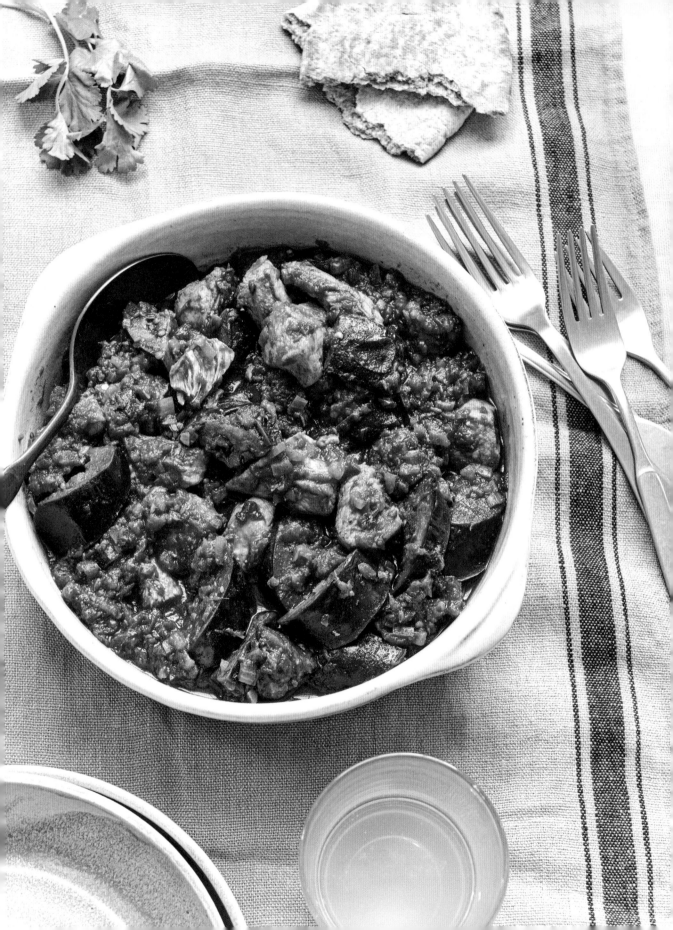

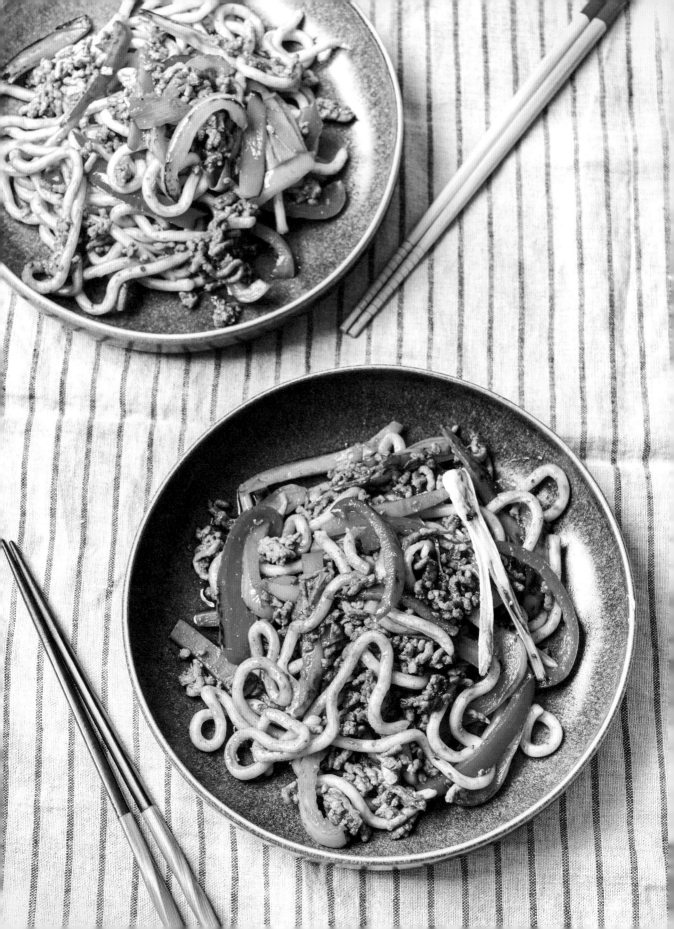

STIR-FRIED CHAR SIU PORK WITH UDON NOODLES

SERVES 4
PREP TIME: 10 MINUTES
COOK TIME: 25 MINUTES

spray oil

250g (9oz) lean minced pork (less than 5 per cent fat)

2 garlic cloves, crushed

5cm (2 inch) piece of fresh root ginger, peeled and finely grated

6 spring onions, sliced

2 carrots, cut into thin strips or julienned

1 red pepper, deseeded and cut into thin strips

1 yellow pepper, deseeded and cut into thin strips

450g (1lb) straight-to-wok udon noodles

FOR THE SAUCE

2 tablespoons tomato purée

2 tablespoons hoisin sauce

2 tablespoons dark soy sauce

1 tablespoon honey

1 tablespoon rice wine

1 teaspoon Chinese 5-spice

Inspired by the delicious flavours of Chinese char siu pork, this quick stir-fry is a perfect easy Friday night fakeaway.

1   Make up the sauce in a small bowl by mixing together all the ingredients.

2   Spray a sauté pan with oil and set over a medium heat. Fry the minced pork, garlic, ginger and spring onions for 10 minutes, breaking up clumps in the minced meat as it cooks.

3   Add the carrot and pepper strips and stir-fry for another 5 minutes.

4   Pour in the sauce and stir-fry for another 10 minutes.

5   Add the pre-cooked noodles to the char-siu pork and stir well to fully combine. Divide between 4 bowls and serve.

PER SERVING
CALORIES 370
FAT 4.5G
SAT FAT 1G
CARBS 55G
SUGARS 16G
FIBRE 7.3G
PROTEIN 23G
SALT 1.7G

SWEET & SOUR PORK

SERVES 4
PREP TIME: 10 MINUTES
COOK TIME: 30 MINUTES

2 garlic cloves, halved

3cm (1¼ inch) piece of root ginger, peeled and roughly chopped

2 tablespoons tomato purée

2 tablespoons rice vinegar

4 tablespoons light soy sauce

1 tablespoon honey

432g (15oz) can of pineapple chunks in juice, drained

1 teaspoon sesame oil

1 red onion, chopped

1 pork tenderloin (about 500g / 1lb 2oz), thinly sliced

2 red, yellow or orange peppers, deseeded and chopped

Here's a great way to make a lip-smacking sweet-and-sour sauce without overdoing the sugar that you'll find in many recipes. A small amount of honey and canned pineapple are all the sweetness you need. Serve with noodles or rice and any extra green vegetables that you fancy.

1   To make the sauce, put the garlic and ginger in a mini chopper or blender with the tomato purée, rice vinegar, soy sauce, honey and pineapple chunks with their juice and blend until smooth.

2   Put the sesame oil in a sauté pan over a high heat and stir-fry the onion for about 2 minutes, then add the pork and peppers and reduce the heat to medium. Stir-fry for 10 minutes.

3   Add the sauce from the mini chopper or blender to the pan and simmer for 15 minutes. Serve with the side dishes of your choice.

PER SERVING
CALORIES 327
FAT 5.3G
SAT FAT 2G
CARBS 25G
SUGARS 23G
FIBRE 3.9G
PROTEIN 42G
SALT 2.2G

Note

You can swap out the pork for chicken, or, for a vegetarian version fry some cubes of firm tofu instead of pork.

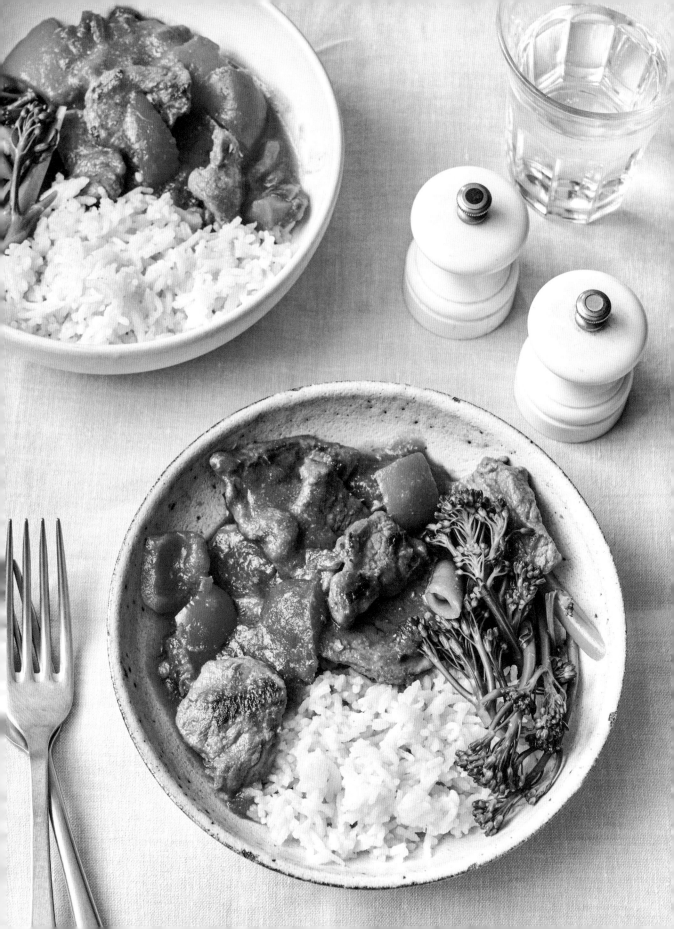

SPICED LAMB & AUBERGINE RICE WITH MINTY YOGURT

SERVES 4
PREP TIME: 10 MINUTES
COOK TIME: 40 MINUTES

spray oil

1 red onion, finely chopped

250g (9oz) reduced-fat minced lamb (less than 10 per cent fat, if possible)

1 large aubergine, chopped into 1cm (½ inch) pieces

2 garlic cloves, crushed

1 tablespoon Ras El Hanout Spice Mix (see page 226 for homemade)

200g (7oz) basmati rice

200g (7oz) tomato passata

450ml (16fl oz) hot chicken stock

1 tablespoon honey

1 teaspoon dried parsley

½ teaspoon coarse ground salt

large handful of mint leaves, finely chopped, some reserved to garnish

125g (4½oz) fat-free Greek yogurt

1 lemon, cut into wedges, to serve

Using minced lamb is a great way of getting the meat's flavour into a meal in a more budget-friendly way. Supplementing lamb with tender aubergine in this dish makes for a tasty and special one-pan Friday meal.

1 Spray a sauté pan, which has a lid, with oil and place over a medium heat. Stir-fry the onion for 3 minutes, then add the minced lamb. Stir-fry this for a further 5 minutes, breaking up any large clumps with the spoon.

2 Add the cubes of aubergine, increase the heat and stir-fry for 3 minutes. Now add the garlic and ras el hanout spice mix and stir everything together.

3 Tip in the rice, passata, stock, honey, dried parsley and salt and stir well. Increase the heat until the dish is bubbling, then reduce it to a gentle simmer. Pop the lid on the pan and allow to simmer gently for 15 minutes, stirring every now and again.

4 Remove the pan from the heat, but leave the lid on, and allow to rest for 10 minutes. After this time the rice should be tender.

5 Meanwhile, make the minty yogurt by simply stirring the chopped fresh mint into the yogurt with a pinch of salt.

6 Divide the rice between 4 bowls, and serve with some of the minty yogurt on top and scattered with the reserved mint leaves, and with a lemon wedge on the side.

PER SERVING
CALORIES 402
FAT 7.3G
SAT FAT 3G
CARBS 54G
SUGARS 14G
FIBRE 5.5G
PROTEIN 25G
SALT 1.7G

Note

To make this vegetarian, simply replace the minced lamb with another large aubergine, or a couple of chopped courgettes or peppers, and replace the chicken stock with vegetable stock.

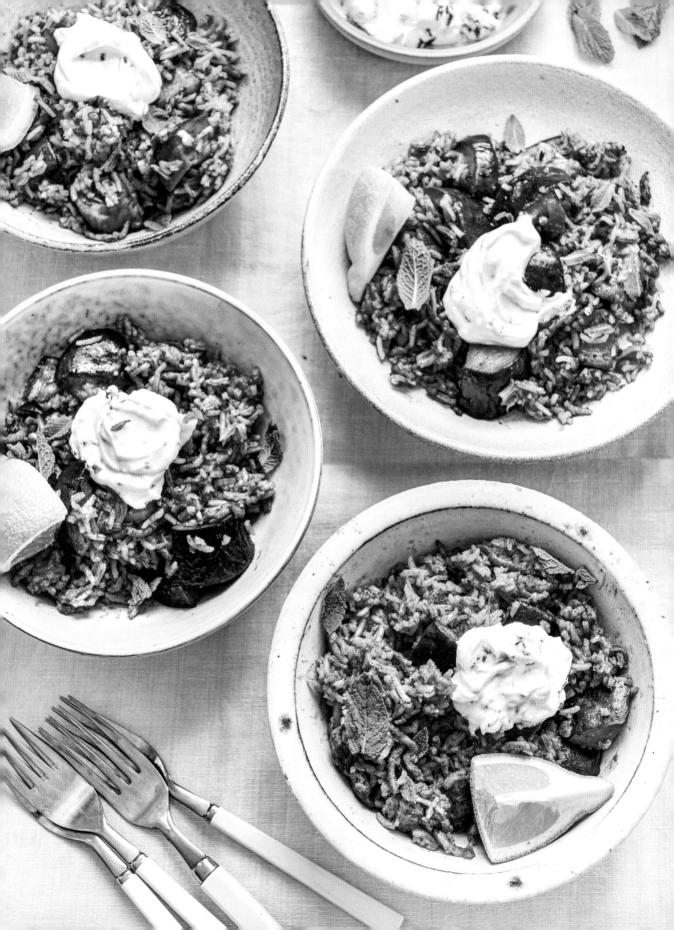

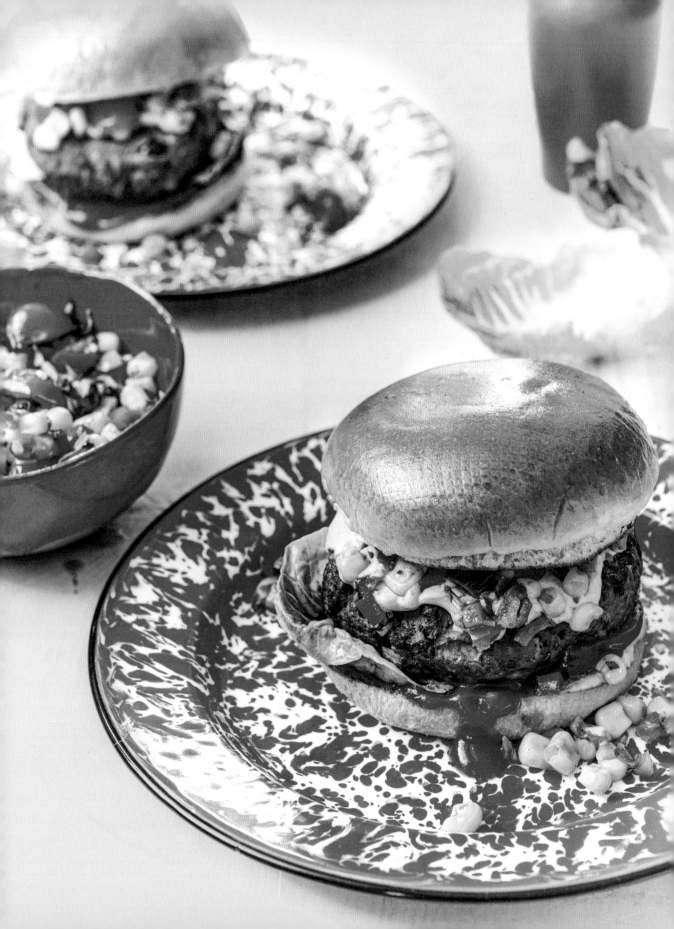

BEEF & BLACK BEAN BURGERS WITH HOT CORN SALSA

FOR THE BURGERS

1 red onion, quartered

1 medium carrot, roughly chopped

1 garlic clove

400g (14oz) can of black beans in water, drained

1 teaspoon dried oregano

½ teaspoon coarse ground salt

½ teaspoon ground cumin

1 tablespoon tomato purée

250g (9oz) lean minced beef

spray oil

4 brioche-style burger buns

FOR THE HOT CORN SALSA

200g (7oz) can of sweetcorn

1 red pepper, finely chopped

1 red onion, finely chopped

150g (5½oz) cherry tomatoes, quartered

handful of coriander leaves and stems, finely chopped

juice of 1 lime

½ teaspoon salt

1 tablespoon finely chopped pickled jalapeños (optional)

OPTIONAL EXTRAS

cheese slices, pickles, pickled jalapeños, mustard, ketchup, lettuce, tomato slices

I love a good, hearty burger, and it is possible to get the satisfaction of a beef burger while cutting down on the meat and adding nutritious and tasty black beans. We have burgers as an occasional treat, so when we do, we usually buy the buttery brioche-style buns, but these can easily be replaced with a wholemeal bread bun for a healthier alternative.

1   Preheat the oven to 210°C/190°C fan (410°F), Gas Mark 6½.

2   In a food processor, whizz together the onion, carrot and garlic for the burgers until they are very finely chopped. Add the black beans, oregano, salt and cumin and pulse to chop them up a little, but don't completely blend: you want to keep a bit of texture. Add the tomato purée and minced beef, then pulse again a couple of times just to bring the mixture together, but you don't want to whizz too much and end up with a paste.

3   Divide the burger mixture into 4 even parts and shape into 4 burgers with your hands, compacting the mixture as much as possible.

4   Line a baking tray with nonstick baking paper and place the burgers on the paper. Spray with oil and bake for 20 minutes, turning them over (carefully so as not to break them) halfway through cooking.

5   Meanwhile, prepare the hot corn salsa. Spray a frying pan with oil. Drain the sweetcorn and fry over a high heat for 5 minutes, to get some of it a little charred and browned. Stir in the red pepper, onion and cherry tomatoes and stir-fry for 2 more minutes. Remove from the heat, spoon into a bowl, then mix in the coriander leaves and stems, lime juice, salt and jalapeños, if using.

6   When the burgers have a couple of minutes of cooking time left, slice the brioche buns in half, lay them on a large baking tray and pop them in the oven to lightly toast for a couple of minutes.

7   Make up the burgers to taste with whatever extras you prefer and serve with the hot corn salsa.

PER SERVING

CALORIES 404

FAT 7.8G

SAT FAT 2.8G

CARBS 50G

SUGARS 16G

FIBRE 9.3G

PROTEIN 26G

SALT 1.9G

Note

If you have bought a 500g (1lb 2oz) pack of minced beef, you can use the other half to make a Bolognese sauce (see page 180) and stretch it out to cover 2 meals. For the Bolognese, simply use the remaining 250g (9oz) minced meat and a 400g (14oz) can of green lentils, drained. Or use the remaining meat for my Barbecue Beefaroni (see page 78).

CHILLI-PEANUT BEEF & NOODLES

SERVES 4
PREP TIME: 10 MINUTES
COOK TIME: 15 MINUTES

1 teaspoon sesame oil

500g (1lb 2oz) lean minced beef (less than 5 per cent fat)

2 garlic cloves, crushed

5cm (2 inch) piece of fresh root ginger, peeled and very finely chopped or grated

1 bunch of spring onions, sliced

200g (7oz) baby button mushrooms, halved

1 carrot, grated

1 teaspoon chilli flakes

2 tablespoons dark soy sauce

2 tablespoons crunchy peanut butter

1 tablespoon honey

200g (7oz) dried egg noodles

coriander leaves, chopped, to serve

Spice up minced beef with a deliciously moreish chilli-peanut dressing. This doesn't have a sauce, but you will discover that frying the meat quite dry really infuses the flavours into the beef.

1 Heat the sesame oil in a sauté pan over a high heat, then add the minced beef and fry for 5 minutes, stirring and breaking up any clumps as it cooks.

2 Add the garlic, ginger, spring onions, mushrooms, carrot and chilli flakes and stir-fry over a medium heat for another 5 minutes.

3 Now pour in the soy sauce, add the peanut butter and honey, stir well to combine and cook over a medium heat for 5 minutes, stirring every now and again as it cooks to prevent it sticking to the pan.

4 Meanwhile, cook the noodles according to the packet instructions.

5 Serve the chilli-peanut beef over the noodles, scattered with chopped coriander.

PER SERVING
CALORIES 503
FAT 14G
SAT FAT 3.9G
CARBS 43G
SUGARS 8.1G
FIBRE 4.9G
PROTEIN 50G
SALT 2.1G

Note

If you want some extra vegetables alongside the beef and noodles, it pairs well with fresh, crunchy salads and veg. Try sliced Little Gem lettuces, more grated carrot, finely sliced radishes, crunchy cucumber or chopped peppers.

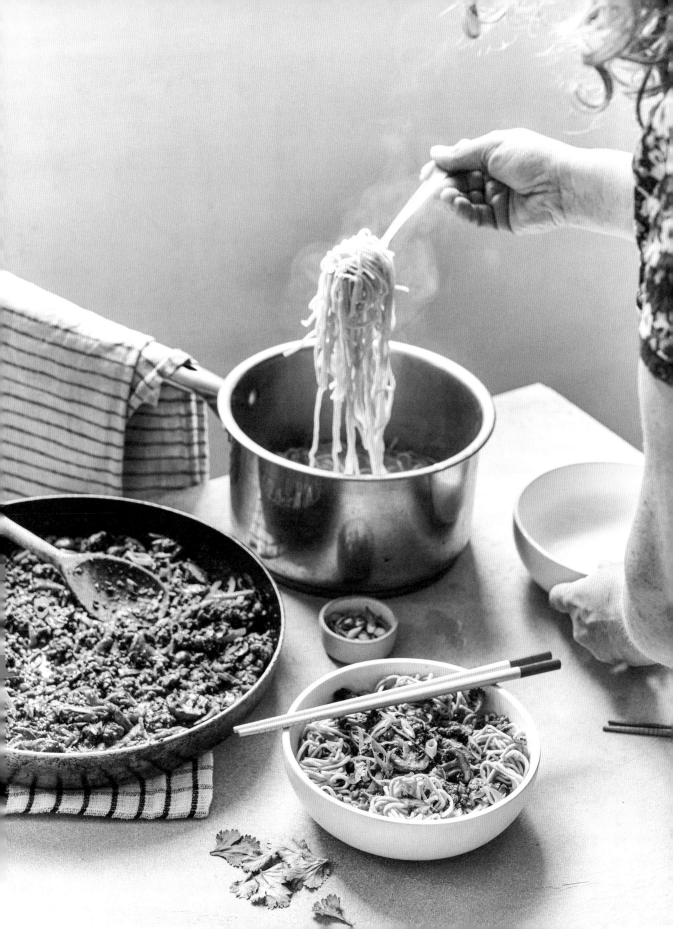

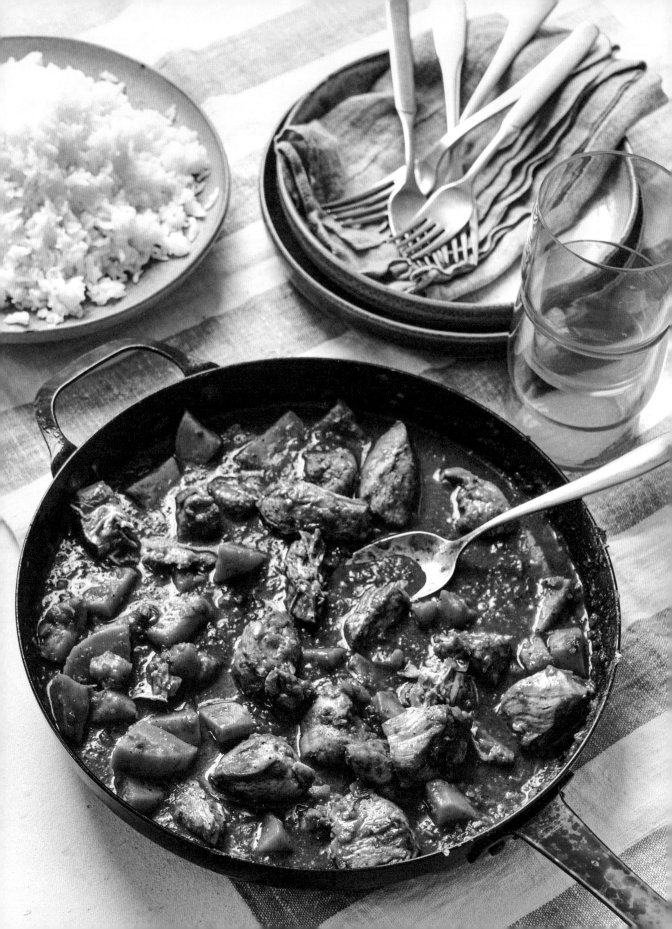

CHICKEN & SWEET POTATO VINDALOO

SERVES 4
PREP TIME: 15 MINUTES
COOK TIME: 50 MINUTES

spray oil

1 large onion, chopped

5cm (2 inch) piece of fresh root ginger, peeled and roughly chopped

5 garlic cloves, peeled

4 tablespoons white wine vinegar

1 tablespoon garam masala

2 teaspoons chilli flakes

1 teaspoon soft brown sugar

1 teaspoon ground coriander

1 teaspoon coarse ground salt

½ teaspoon ground fenugreek

½ teaspoon mustard powder

½ teaspoon ground turmeric

¼ teaspoon freshly ground black pepper

4 chicken breasts (total weight about 600g / 1lb 5oz), cut into chunks

2 tablespoons tomato purée

500ml (18fl oz) hot chicken stock

1–2 large sweet potatoes (total weight about 500g / 1lb 2oz), chopped

The first time I tried vindaloo was at an Indian cookery evening held at my secondary school in the early 1990s, when the mum of one of my classmates came in and demonstrated a few recipes, which I still use to this day. My mum and I actually won the chicken vindaloo in the raffle! I tried a piece of the chicken in the car on the way home and it was the hottest thing I had ever eaten, but I absolutely loved it. This vindaloo is based on that recipe (and sadly I don't remember the original cook's details to give her credit), though I have made a few adjustments over the years, adding sweet potato to bulk out the chicken. I serve this with basmati rice.

1   Spray a sauté pan with oil, place over a medium heat and fry the onion for 8 minutes. Place it in a mini chopper or food processor with the ginger, garlic and 3 tablespoons water and blend into a paste.

2   In a small bowl, mix the vinegar, garam masala, chilli flakes, sugar, coriander, salt, fenugreek, mustard powder, turmeric and black pepper.

3   Add the chicken to the sauté pan, and stir-fry for 5 minutes, then add the garlic and ginger paste and stir-fry for 2 more minutes. Add the vinegar and spice mix and the tomato purée and stir-fry for another 2 minutes.

4   Pour in the chicken stock, add the sweet potato, then simmer gently for 30 minutes, stirring occasionally. Serve once the sweet potato is tender and the curry fragrant.

PER SERVING
CALORIES 352
FAT 3.2G
SAT FAT 0.8G
CARBS 35G
SUGARS 13G
FIBRE 5.6G
PROTEIN 42G
SALT 2.3G

Note

I have been quite restrained with the amount of chilli in this, but if you love a fiery heat, please do add 1–2 green finger chillies to blend into the ginger and garlic paste.

- ✔ CHICKEN AND SWEET POTATO SATAY HOTPOT
- ✔ CREAMY CHICKEN CHANGEZI CURRY
- ✔ HARISSA AND COCONUT BRAISED CHICKEN
- ✔ TERIYAKI CHICKEN BALLS
- ✔ CHICKEN TAGINE
- ✔ JUICY PULLED CHICKEN
- ✔ PORK GYOZA
- ✔ CHORIZO, CHILLI AND ROASTED PEPPER ORZO
- ✔ MAC 'N' CHEESE LASAGNE
- ✔ EVERYTHING SEASONED DOUGH BALLS

6

Sumptuous Saturday

CHICKEN & SWEET POTATO SATAY HOTPOT

SERVES 4
PREP TIME: 5 MINUTES
COOK TIME: 55 MINUTES

spray oil

1 onion, chopped

3 chicken breasts (about 450g / 1lb), cut into chunks

2 garlic cloves, crushed

500ml (18fl oz) hot chicken stock

4 tablespoons peanut butter, smooth or crunchy

3 tablespoons tomato purée

2 tablespoons dark soy sauce

1 tablespoon honey

1 teaspoon chilli powder, mild or hot, to taste

1 teaspoon ground coriander

juice of 1 lemon

500g (1lb 2oz) sweet potato, cut into chunks

coriander leaves or sliced spring onions, to serve

Thick, rich satay sauce with tender chicken and sweet potato makes for a delicious treat meal. Satay-style sauces have always been one of my favourite indulgences, and here you get plenty of delicious flavour without an excess of sugar and using only a small amount of peanut butter. I usually serve this simply with basmati rice and green vegetables, but it also works well with noodles.

1   Preheat the oven to 200°C/180°C fan (400°F), Gas Mark 6.

2   Spray a flameproof casserole dish, which has a lid, with oil and place over a medium-high heat. (I use a nonstick hob-to-oven casserole.) Fry the onion for 5 minutes to soften it, then add the chicken chunks. Stir-fry the chicken for 3–4 minutes to seal it, then stir in the garlic and fry for another minute.

3   Pour in the hot chicken stock, then add the peanut butter, tomato purée, soy sauce, honey, chilli powder, ground coriander, lemon juice and sweet potato.

4   Keep over a medium heat while you stir all the ingredients together to make sure that the peanut butter has melted into the sauce.

5   Pop the lid on the pan and place it on the middle shelf of the oven for 40 minutes. Serve scattered with the coriander leaves or spring onions.

PER SERVING
CALORIES 430
FAT 13G
SAT FAT 2.5G
CARBS 36G
SUGARS 16G
FIBRE 6.1G
PROTEIN 38G
SALT 2.3G

Note

For a vegetarian version you could use a mix of other vegetables instead of the chicken, such as carrots, regular potatoes, cauliflower, mushrooms, squash, corn and beetroot. Make sure that you are using a vegetarian soy sauce and replace the chicken stock with vegetable stock.

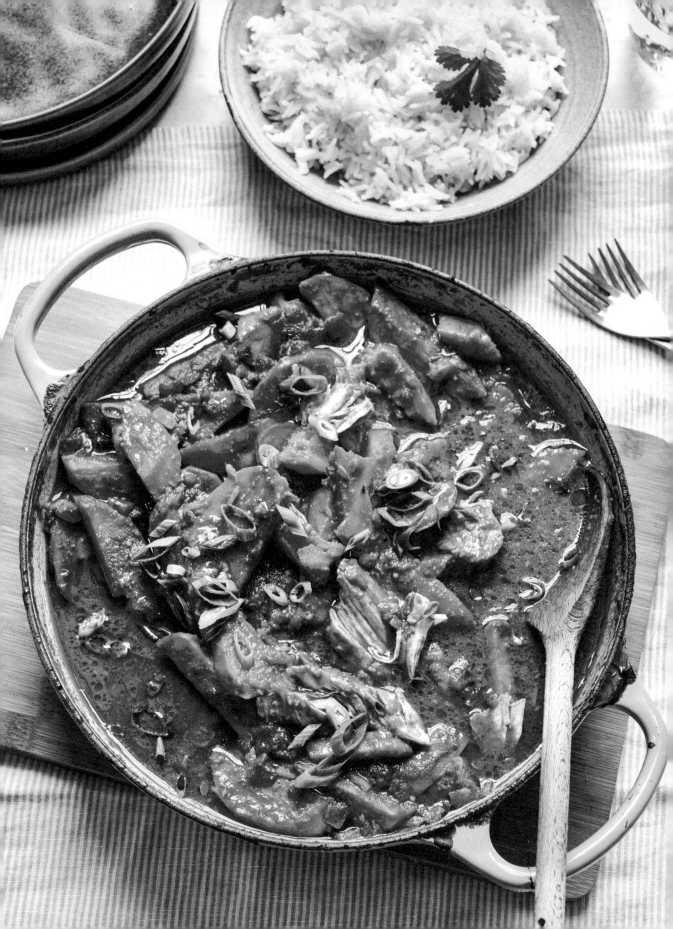

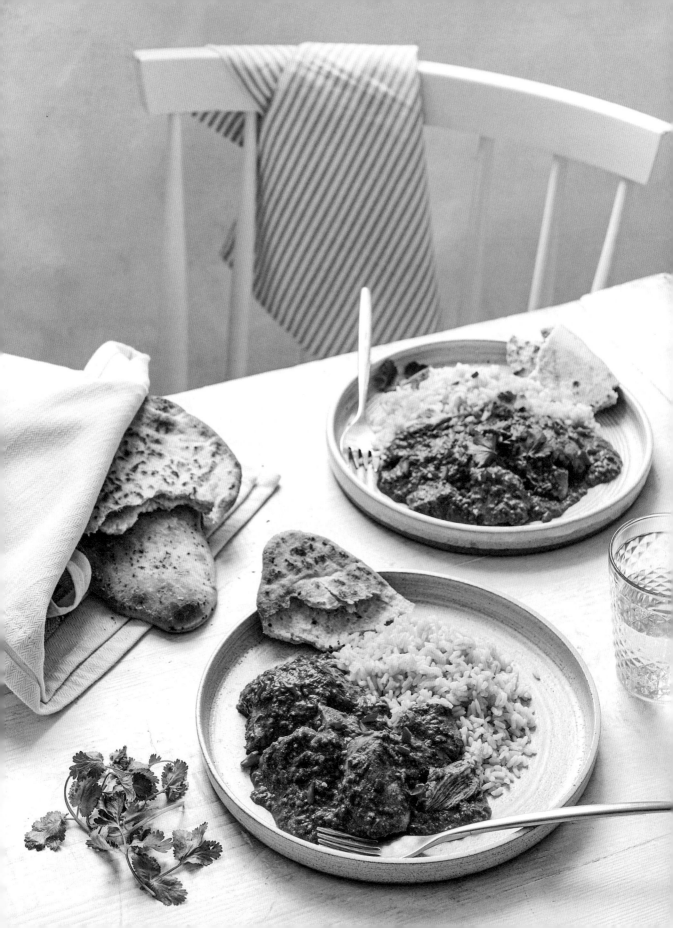

CREAMY CHICKEN CHANGEZI CURRY

SERVES 4
PREP TIME: 10 MINUTES
COOK TIME: 40 MINUTES

3–4 chicken breasts (around 600g / 1lb 5oz), cut into chunks
salt and pepper
coriander leaves, to serve

FOR THE MARINADE

150g (5½oz) fat-free Greek yogurt
2.5cm (1 inch) piece of fresh root ginger, peeled and finely grated
3 garlic cloves, crushed or finely grated
1 red chilli, deseeded and finely chopped
juice of ½ lemon

FOR THE SAUCE

1 tablespoon butter
2 red onions, sliced
15 whole cashew nuts (about 50g / 1¾oz)
4 tablespoons tomato purée
1 teaspoon ground coriander
1 teaspoon ground turmeric
1 teaspoon mild chilli powder
½ teaspoon coarse ground salt
250ml (9fl oz) semi-skimmed milk
4 tablespoons single cream

If you love a cream- or butter-based curry – such as chicken tikka masala or makhani – then this one is for you. It has a decadent-tasting sauce, but only uses a small amount of cream and butter and gets the rest of its creaminess from blended cashews, milk and yogurt. My version is simple to make; blending up the onions and cashews is probably the faffiest bit and, in reality, that only takes a few minutes. I absolutely recommend this as a Saturday night treat that won't leave you wishing you'd ordered a takeaway! I like to serve this with basmati rice and naan.

1   In a large bowl, mix up the marinade ingredients, stir in the chicken chunks, season with salt and pepper, then set aside.

2   Melt the butter in a sauté pan, add the sliced onions and cashew nuts and fry for 10 minutes, stirring every now and again. Spoon the fried onions and cashews into a mini chopper and blend them up into a paste.

3   Pour the chicken and yogurt mixture into the sauté pan and fry for 10 minutes over a medium-high heat, stirring regularly.

4   Reduce the heat slightly and add the onion and cashew paste, tomato purée, ground coriander, turmeric, chilli powder and salt. Pour in the milk: don't worry if it splits (becomes grainy looking) here, as it won't cause an issue with the final dish. Stir everything together well and simmer gently for 15 minutes.

5   Stir through the single cream and garam masala and serve scattered with coriander leaves.

PER SERVING
CALORIES 401
FAT 15G
SAT FAT 6.2G
CARBS 17G
SUGARS 12G
FIBRE 2.1G
PROTEIN 47G
SALT 1.3G

Note

I find that grating ginger is the easiest way to prepare it for this type of dish. A handy way to ensure that your ginger is both available and easy to grate is to freeze it. Simply cut a fresh root of ginger up into useable sizes (most of my recipes call for a piece about 2–3cm / 1 inch) and pop it into a freezer-safe sealed bag or storage container. Then, whenever a recipe calls for fresh root ginger, you can just take a piece out of the freezer, peel it with a peeler or teaspoon, then grate it directly from frozen.

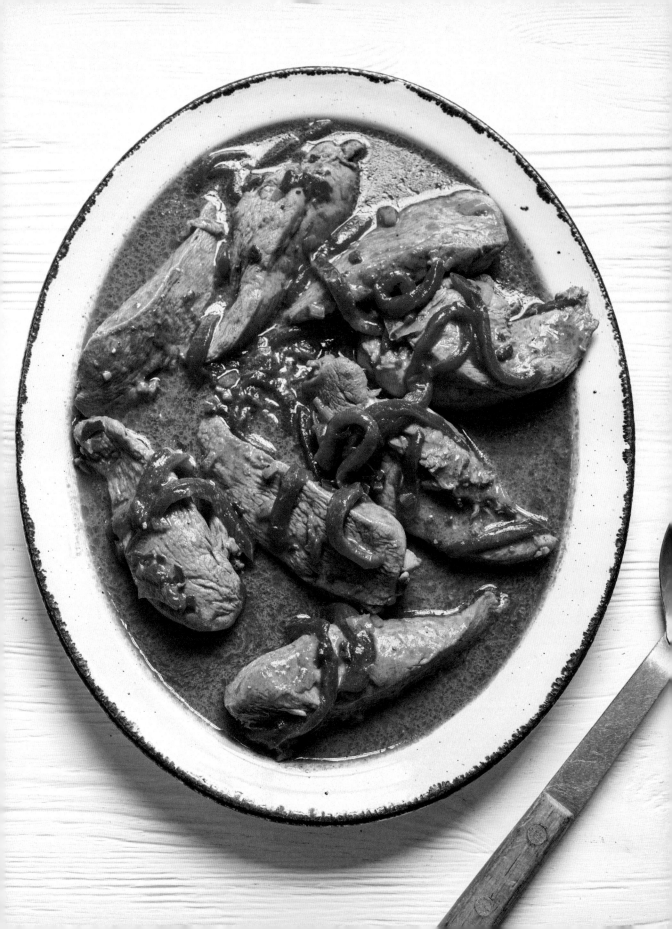

HARISSA & COCONUT BRAISED CHICKEN

SERVES 4
PREP TIME: 10 MINUTES
COOK TIME: 35 MINUTES

spray oil

1 onion, chopped

2 garlic cloves, crushed

2 tablespoons tomato purée

50ml (2fl oz) water

400g (14oz) can of light coconut milk

1 tablespoon harissa paste

½ teaspoon coarse ground salt

handful of basil leaves, plus more to serve

4 small skinless chicken breasts (total weight about 600g / 1lb 5oz), halved lengthways from the top down

2 roasted red peppers from a jar, thinly sliced

240g (8½oz) jasmine rice

Tender chicken breast, braised in a creamy coconut and harissa sauce, is an indulgent-tasting meal which is also quick and easy to pull together. I serve this with jasmine rice and steamed greens such as broccoli, crisp sugar snaps or asparagus.

1   Spray a sauté pan, which has a lid, with oil and place over a medium heat. Fry the onion for 10 minutes until soft. Add the garlic and tomato purée and stir-fry for 2 minutes, then add the water and deglaze the pan by using a wooden spoon to stir any stuck on bits into the liquid.

2   Add the coconut milk, harissa, salt and basil leaves, stir, then add the chicken breast pieces and the sliced peppers. Pop a lid on the pan and simmer for 20 minutes.

3   When 15 minutes are remaining on the chicken, put the jasmine rice on to cook (see page 118 for cooking instructions).

4   For the final 3 minutes of chicken cooking time, put the broccoli florets into a large pan of boiling water, simmer for 3 minutes, then drain.

5   Serve the chicken and sauce over the rice with your favourite green vegetables on the side.

PER SERVING

CALORIES 523

FAT 10G

SAT FAT 6.9G

CARBS 59G

SUGARS 8.8G

FIBRE 5.7G

PROTEIN 46G

SALT 0.93G

TERIYAKI CHICKEN BALLS

SERVES 4
PREP TIME: 15 MINUTES
COOK TIME: 20 MINUTES

400g (14oz) can of pinto beans, in water, drained and rinsed

500g (1lb 2oz) minced chicken (less than 5 per cent fat)

2 garlic cloves, crushed

3cm (1¼ inch) piece of fresh root ginger, peeled and finely grated

1 tablespoon light soy sauce

4 spring onions, finely chopped, plus 2 more to serve

2 teaspoons sesame oil

4 tablespoons teriyaki sauce

1 tablespoon sesame seeds, to serve

A different take on meatballs, these juicy chicken numbers are sticky and glazed with teriyaki. You can either make your own teriyaki sauce (see page 227) or use a shop-bought version (but make sure you pick up teriyaki *sauce*, which has a thick and gloopy consistency, rather than teriyaki *marinade*, which has the consistency of soy sauce). Serve these meatballs over rice or noodles with greens: edamame beans and sugar snaps work well.

1   Make the chicken meatballs. Place the pinto beans in a large mixing bowl and mash them with a potato masher until they are roughly mashed.

2   Add the minced chicken, garlic, ginger, soy sauce and spring onions, then use a metal spoon to thoroughly mix everything together. Use your hands to shape the mixture into 20 meatballs.

3   Heat a frying pan with the sesame oil over a medium-low heat. Add the chicken meatballs and fry for 12–14 minutes, mixing and shuffling them around with a spatula to ensure they are evenly cooked on all sides. (You can check they are fully cooked through with a meat thermometer: they should have an internal temperature of at least 75°C / 167°F.)

4   Drizzle the teriyaki sauce all over the cooked meatballs and stir-fry them over a high heat for a final 2 minutes to coat all the meatballs in sauce.

5   Serve scattered with sesame seeds and sliced spring onions.

PER SERVING
CALORIES 266
FAT 9.2G
SAT FAT 2G
CARBS 13G
SUGARS 3.8G
FIBRE 4.2G
PROTEIN 31G
SALT 2.5G

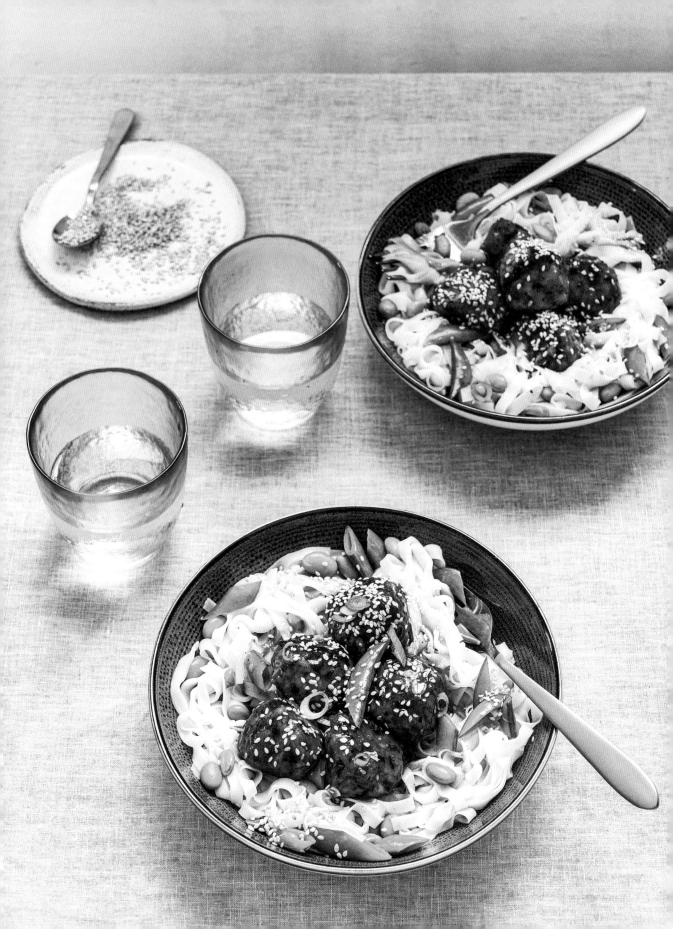

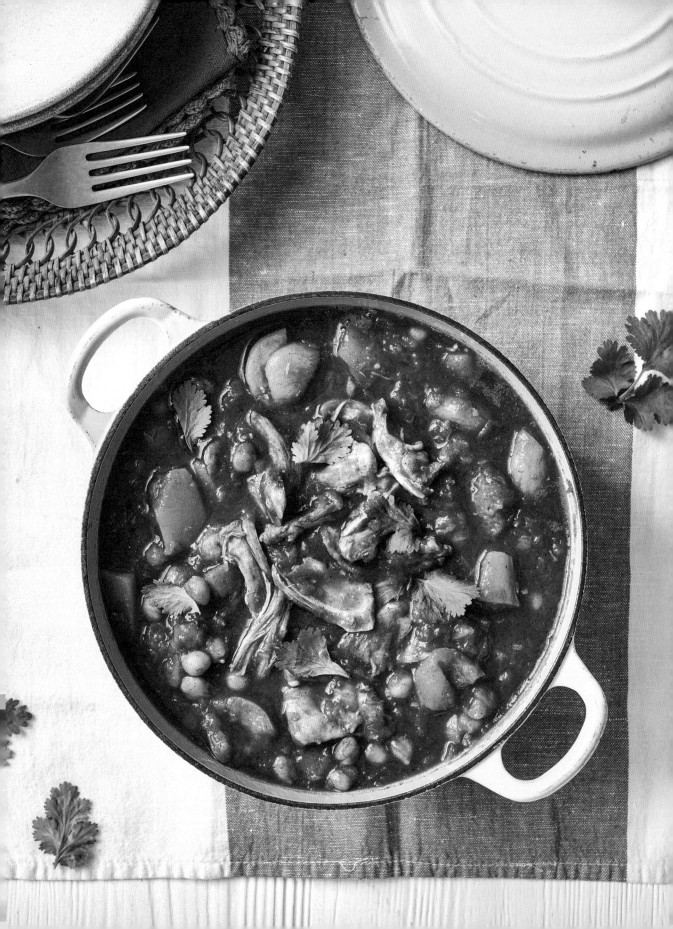

CHICKEN TAGINE

SERVES 6
PREP TIME: 15 MINUTES
COOK TIME: 40 MINUTES

1 tablespoon olive oil

8 skinless chicken thigh fillets

2 onions, chopped

3 garlic cloves, crushed

2 tablespoons Ras El Hanout Spice Mix (see page 226 for homemade)

2 tablespoons tomato purée

400g (14oz) can of chopped tomatoes

2 x 400g (14oz) cans of chickpeas in water, drained and rinsed

120g (4¼oz) dried apricots, cut into quarters

750ml (1 pint 6fl oz) hot chicken stock

500g (1lb 2oz) fresh or frozen butternut squash, cut into cubes

½ teaspoon coarse ground salt

finely grated zest and juice of 1 lemon

handful of coriander leaves, chopped, to serve

A tagine is a classic North African stew made with meat or fish and vegetables gently braised in a fragrantly spiced sauce. It's called a tagine after the special type of pot used to cook it, which has a funnel-shaped lid. As many of us won't have a tagine at home, this version is simply made in a casserole dish, but the flavours and ingredients are inspired by the traditional version. You'll find this a great meal for serving up to friends and family, or simply freezing leftovers for another day. You can serve it on its own, with flatbreads to mop up the sauce, or alongside rice. You may want extra vegetables on the side: this works well alongside a red cabbage salad, freshly sliced cucumber, grilled aubergines, roasted carrots or any steamed green vegetables.

1   Heat the oil in a large casserole pot over a medium heat. Fry the chicken and onions in the olive oil for 8 minutes, stirring occasionally. Add the garlic and stir-fry for another minute. Add the ras el hanout and tomato purée and stir-fry for another minute.

2   Tip in the chopped tomatoes, chickpeas, apricots, chicken stock, butternut squash and salt and stir everything together. Bring to the boil, then reduce the heat and simmer for 25 minutes.

3   Remove the chicken from the pan to a chopping board and roughly slice each thigh into strips, then return the meat to the pan and stir it in.

4   Add the lemon zest and juice and stir through. Serve scattered with coriander.

Note

PER SERVING
CALORIES 459
FAT 10G
SAT FAT 2.1G
CARBS 38G
SUGARS 21G
FIBRE 14G
PROTEIN 46G
SALT 2G

>   If you wish to make a vegetarian version of this, replace the chicken with vegetables such as chopped aubergines, peppers, green beans, tomatoes, cauliflower, carrots and regular potatoes or sweet potatoes. Just add the vegetables in step 2, replacing the chicken stock with vegetable stock.

>   If you can't get hold of ras el hanout, or don't have time to make my suggested spice mix (see page 226), then use this simplified recipe. In a small bowl, mix together 1 teaspoon ground cinnamon, 1 teaspoon ground cumin, 1 teaspoon ground turmeric, ½ teaspoon chilli powder and 1 teaspoon sweet paprika.

JUICY PULLED CHICKEN

SERVES 6
PREP TIME: 5 MINUTES
COOK TIME: 45 MINUTES

12 skinless chicken thigh fillets

1 onion, sliced

3 garlic cloves, crushed

2 teaspoons ground cumin

1 bay leaf

1 teaspoon coarse ground salt

½ teaspoon freshly ground black pepper

This delicious pulled chicken can be served in numerous ways. By braising the chicken, it remains tender, juicy and full of flavour. It's the perfect base for many different meals – see below for some of my favourite suggestions. Don't throw away the sauce that remains in the pan at the end of cooking, as it makes an excellent soup base: just store it in an airtight container in the refrigerator or the freezer to add next time you are making soup.

1   Put all the ingredients into a large pan and cover with water, but only use as much water as you need for your pan. You don't want excess liquid here, as you will be reducing it down at the end.

2   Place over a high heat and bring to the boil, then reduce the heat slightly and allow it to simmer for 30 minutes. Remove the chicken from the pan into a large bowl, or plastic storage tub if you are keeping it for later.

3   Replace the saucepan and liquid over a high heat and allow to bubble vigorously for 10 minutes to reduce the liquid and concentrate the remaining flavours.

4   Meanwhile, use 2 forks to shred the chicken apart as much as you can and place it in a shallow dish.

5   Remove the pan from the heat and pour about 200ml (7fl oz) of the remaining liquid over the shredded chicken. This will help keep it moist and flavoursome. Mix it through until the meat has absorbed the liquid.

Note

Here are some ideas of how you can use pulled chicken:

> For tacos or burritos: use as a filling and serve it up in tortillas with shredded lettuce, chopped tomatoes, cheese, refried beans and salsa.
> With a Mexican-style salsa verde: take 1 deseeded and chopped green pepper, 1 tablespoon pickled jalapeños, 1 tablespoon honey, a handful of coriander, the finely grated zest and juice of 1 lime, 1 teaspoon oregano and ½ teaspoon salt and whizz in a blender – the perfect sauce for a pulled chicken burrito.
> In a burger bun with a homemade slaw and barbecue sauce.
> As part of a salad: it's great in both grain-based and green salads, with added extras such as avocado, cucumber and fresh herbs.
> As a filling for quesadillas.
> In a Chinese-style wrap with shredded lettuce, cucumber matchsticks, spring onions and teriyaki sauce (see page 227 for homemade).
> As an addition to pasta with a tomato-based or creamy sauce (see page 88 for Pasta Sauce 3 Ways).

PER SERVING
CALORIES 276
FAT 6.9G
SAT FAT 1.9G
CARBS 2.5G
SUGARS 1.6G
FIBRE 0.7G
PROTEIN 37G
SALT 1.4G

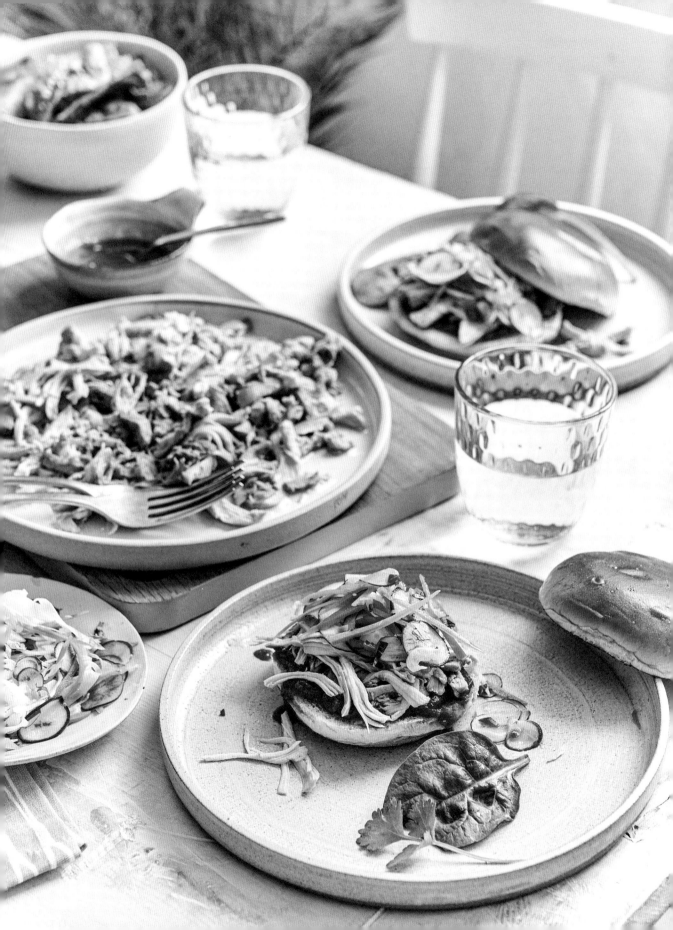

PORK GYOZA

SERVES 4
PREP TIME: 40 MINUTES
COOK TIME: 30 MINUTES

175g (6oz) plain flour, plus more to dust

175ml (6fl oz) boiling water

pinch of salt

300g (10½oz) lean minced pork (less than 5 per cent fat)

2cm (¾ inch) piece of fresh root ginger, peeled and finely grated

3 spring onions, thinly sliced

100g (3½oz) Brussels sprouts, outer leaves and stalks removed, halved and thinly sliced (see note, opposite)

1 tablespoon light soy sauce

2 tablespoons vegetable oil

200ml (7fl oz) cold water

FOR THE DIPPING SAUCE

2 tablespoons light soy sauce

1 tablespoon honey

1 teaspoon rice vinegar

1 teaspoon chilli sauce (optional)

Most of my recipes are straightforward and quick to cook. This one is a little bit more time-consuming, but it makes a lovely meal and is well worth the extra effort. My girls really love gyoza and it's a fun dish to make with kids. The filling is super-simple and only requires mixing up, while rolling out and crimping the gyoza is a great activity for everyone to do together. You can buy frozen gyoza skins, which makes this whole process a lot faster, but I haven't found these to be easily available in supermarkets (other than specialist shops), which is why I tend to make my own. Serve with Sesame Shredded Carrot Salad (see page 215).

1   To make the dough, tip the flour into a bowl, pour in the boiling water, add the pinch of salt and use a table knife to mix them together to start to form a dough. Once the dough has started to form, use your hands to bring it together into a ball.

2   Place the dough on a lightly floured work surface and knead for about 2 minutes, until it is smooth. If you aren't going to use it right away, dust it with a little flour and wrap it in clingfilm until you need it.

3   Now mix up the filling in a large bowl. Simply put in the pork, ginger, spring onions, Brussels sprouts and soy sauce in a bowl and mix well with a wooden spoon, breaking up any clumps in the minced meat.

4   To make the gyoza skins, take the ball of dough and divide it into 8 equal pieces. Now split each piece into 3 equal pieces. You should have 24 fairly uniformly sized small pieces of dough. (You may find it easier to make 2 sausage shapes with the dough, then cut each into 12.)

5   Dust your work surface with flour and keep some on hand to keep your rolling pin and hands dusted to prevent sticking. One at a time, with your hands, roll each piece of dough into a smooth ball, press it down on the work surface with the palm of your hand to form a flat, round disc, then use a rolling pin to roll it into a circle about 9cm in diameter. These do not have to be perfect (mine are always pretty rustic!) but if you want to create a perfect shape, use a 9cm round or fluted cutter to neaten up the edges. Repeat until you have made all the skins. If you are piling them up, make sure you sprinkle a little flour in between them so they don't stick together.

6   Sprinkle flour over 2 dinner plates, ready for you to place the gyoza on before cooking. Have a small bowl of water ready next to you when you start making the gyoza.

7   Take a gyoza skin, put 1 heaped teaspoon of pork filling in the middle, use your finger to dot some water around half the edge of the gyoza skin, then fold it over to make a semicircle, pressing down on the edge to seal it together.

8   You'll find tutorials online for how to pleat gyoza using a traditional method to seal the filling, but I simply seal the edges by using a fork dipped in water to press the edges together for a crimped effect.

9   Place each completed gyoza on a floured plate, but do not pile them on top of each other or they are likely to stick together.

10   To cook the gyoza, pour 1 tablespoon of oil into a sauté pan, which has a lid, use a silicone pastry brush to distribute it evenly over the bottom of the pan, then set the pan over a medium heat and bring it to temperature.

11   Place 12 of the gyoza in the pan, flat sides down, and fry for about 5 minutes. You want the bottoms to turn a golden-brown colour and become a little crispy, but be careful not to burn them. After you have had a little peek at the bottoms to make sure they are golden brown, pour half the measured cold water into the pan, then cover it with the lid.

12   Reduce the heat to just below medium and allow the gyoza to steam for 4 minutes.

13   Remove the lid from the pan, increase the heat to medium once more and allow the remaining water to bubble away until it has all boiled off and just the dumplings remain in the pan. Transfer carefully to a warm plate and keep in a warmed-up oven while you repeat this process with the other 12 dumplings and the remaining oil and measured cold water.

14   To make the dip, place all the ingredients in a small, microwave-safe bowl and microwave for 40 seconds, then stir to mix everything together.

15   Serve the gyoza while fresh and hot, with the dip.

Note

PER SERVING
CALORIES 352
FAT 9.3G
SAT FAT 1.4G
CARBS 39G
SUGARS 6.4G
FIBRE 3.6G
PROTEIN 26G
SALT 1.9G

> I use Brussels sprouts instead of cabbage, because they are so easy to slice very finely and you don't want any big chunks when trying to make up the delicate dumplings. If you prefer to use cabbage, just ensure that you slice it very thinly.

> You can freeze these once cooked and cooled. To do so, line a baking tray with nonstick baking paper and place the dumplings on top, making sure they aren't touching. Transfer to the freezer and allow them to freeze solid (this should take 1–3 hours). Once they have frozen, remove from the freezer and transfer the dumplings into a freezer-safe bag or container.

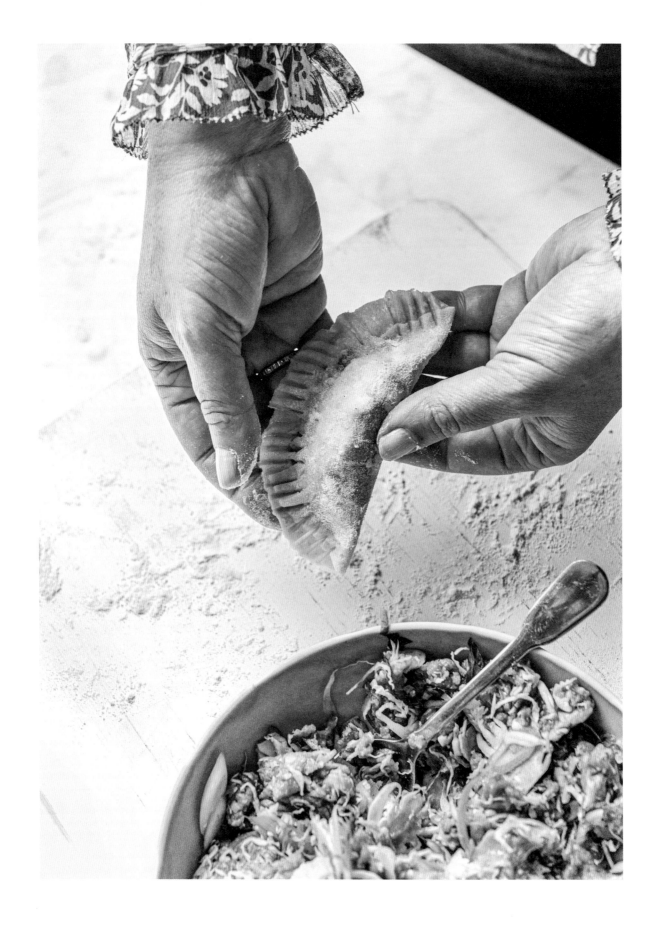

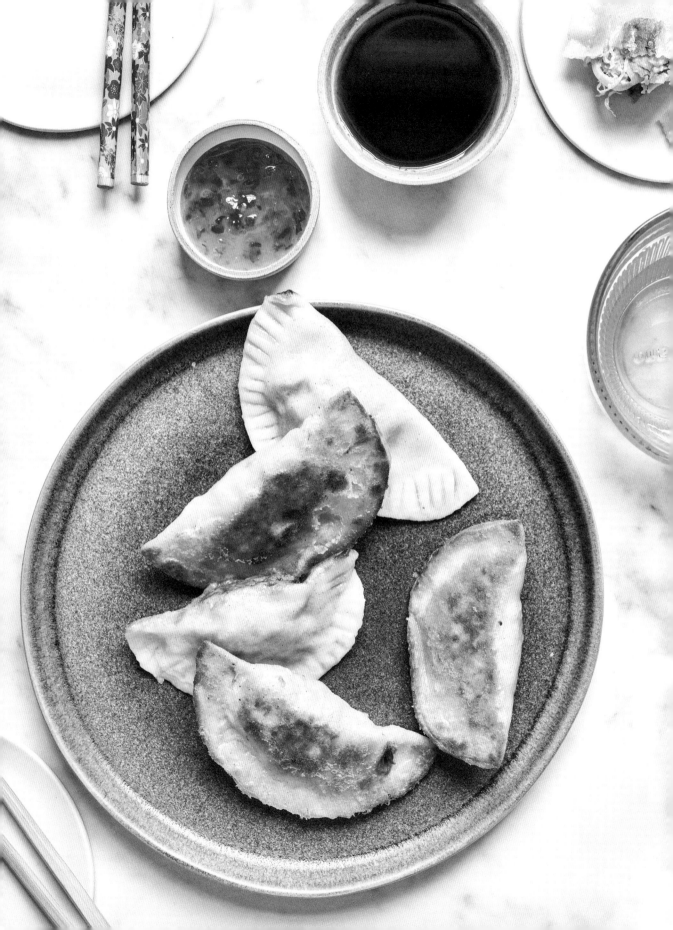

CHORIZO, CHILLI & ROASTED PEPPER ORZO

SERVES 4
PREP TIME: 10 MINUTES
COOK TIME: 30 MINUTES

50g (1¾oz) chorizo, half grated, half very finely chopped

1 red onion, finely chopped

2 garlic cloves, crushed

1 red chilli, deseeded and finely chopped

50g (1¾oz) sundried tomatoes, drained, patted dry with kitchen towel and finely chopped

300g (10½oz) orzo

1 litre (1¾ pints) hot chicken stock

2 whole roasted peppers from a jar, finely sliced

100g (3½oz) frozen spinach

salt and pepper

Parmesan cheese shavings, or Gruyère cheese shavings, to serve (optional)

This is a really satisfying orzo dish, in which a little chorizo goes a long way to giving a beautiful flavour. Grating chorizo is a useful way to maximize the impact that a small amount of the sausage can have on a dish.

1   In a sauté pan, which has a lid, fry the chorizo, onion, garlic and chilli for 10 minutes. There's no need for oil, due to the fat in the chorizo.

2   Stir through the sundried tomatoes and orzo, then add the chicken stock and roasted peppers. Place the lid on the pan and simmer for 15 minutes.

3   Add the spinach, cover and simmer for another 5 minutes.

4   Stir well to distribute the spinach, then season with salt and pepper. Serve with extra cheese shavings, if you like.

PER SERVING
CALORIES 459
FAT 14G
SAT FAT 3.4G
CARBS 59G
SUGARS 8.1G
FIBRE 7.8G
PROTEIN 20G
SALT 2.4G

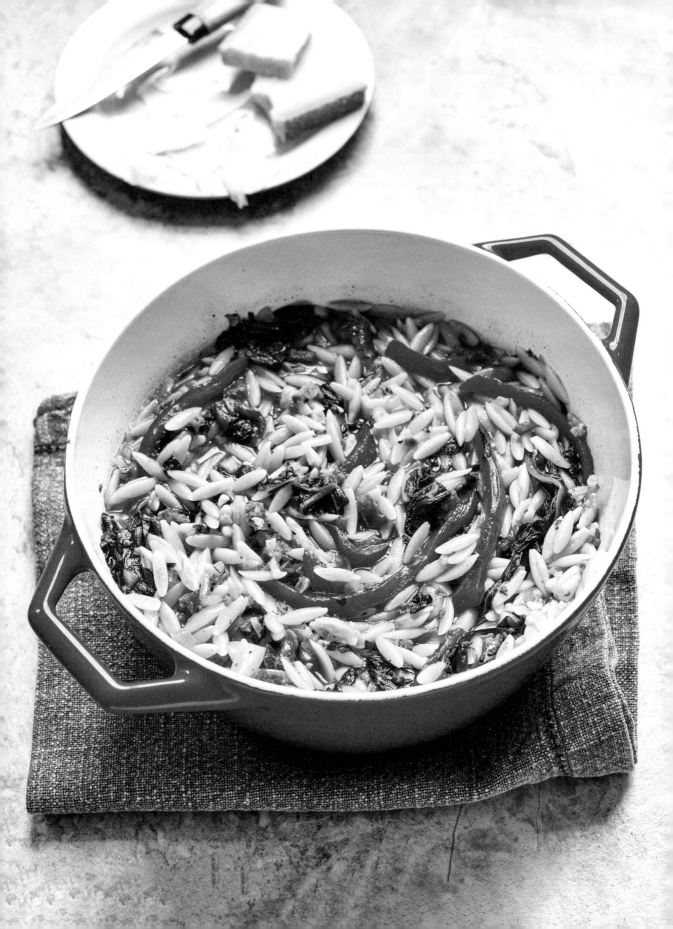

MAC 'N' CHEESE 'LASAGNE'

SERVES 6
PREP TIME: 10 MINUTES
COOK TIME: 45 MINUTES

spray oil

1 onion, chopped

1 carrot, chopped

3 garlic cloves, crushed

500g (1lb 2oz) lean minced beef (less than 5 per cent fat)

500g (1lb 2oz) tomato passata

2 tablespoons tomato purée

1 tablespoon dark soy sauce

1 beef or red wine stock pot, dissolved in a small amount of boiling water

2 teaspoons dried oregano, plus more to sprinkle

1 teaspoon dried basil, plus more to sprinkle

1 teaspoon dried rosemary, plus more to sprinkle

½ teaspoon coarse ground salt

250ml (9fl oz) semi-skimmed milk

500ml (18fl oz) water

300g (10½oz) macaroni

150g (5½oz) reduced-fat cream cheese

60g (2¼oz) mature Cheddar cheese, grated

30g (1oz) Parmesan cheese, finely grated

100g (3½oz) mozzarella cheese, grated or torn into small pieces

salt and pepper

PER SERVING
CALORIES 508
FAT 18G
SAT FAT 10G
CARBS 45G
SUGARS 12G
FIBRE 5G
PROTEIN 37G
SALT 2G

This isn't technically a lasagne, of course, as macaroni is used instead of pasta sheets, but like a lasagne it has layers of rich beef ragu and a four-cheese sauce. My kids much prefer this version as it's easy to eat, while the cheese sauce is much simpler to make than a traditional roux-based bechamel, but still delicious. Serve this with salad or vegetables; it works well with any leftover Peperonata (see page 92).

1   Preheat the oven to 210°C/190°C fan (410°F), Gas Mark 6½.

2   Spray a sauté pan with oil, place over a medium heat and fry the onion for 5 minutes, then add the carrot, garlic and minced beef and stir-fry for another 5 minutes, breaking up any clumps of meat as you stir.

3   Add the passata, tomato purée, soy sauce, stock, oregano, basil, rosemary and salt, then leave to simmer gently, stirring occasionally, while you prepare the macaroni and sauce.

4   In a small saucepan, bring the milk and measured water to the boil, add the macaroni, then reduce the heat to a simmer. Simmer for 10 minutes, stirring occasionally to prevent the macaroni from sticking to the bottom of the pan. After 10 minutes, the macaroni should be cooked through.

5   Add the cream cheese to the pan and stir it through the macaroni until it has melted. Then add half the Cheddar and Parmesan. You want the macaroni mixture to be quite saucy at this point, so if it's looking a little dry, gradually add some freshly boiled water to create more sauce. Season with salt and pepper.

6   In an ovenproof baking dish (I use a rectangular dish measuring 28 x 23cm / 11 x 9 inches), layer in half the meat sauce, then half the macaroni cheese, spreading it around to cover the meat, then repeat the layers. Make sure the macaroni cheese covers the meat, then top it with the mozzarella and remaining Cheddar and Parmesan. Sprinkle over a few extra pinches of the dried herbs, then pop into the oven for 20 minutes, by which time the cheese on top should be golden brown and bubbling and the 'lasagne' will be ready to serve.

It's easy to add extra veggies to this. Try chopped mushrooms, peppers, courgettes or aubergines, frying them into the ragu during step 2. Or layer in baby spinach leaves under the macaroni cheese layers when you assemble the lasagne, or stir some frozen spinach into the macaroni cheese sauce before layering up (though in this case you may need to add some extra water to keep the sauce consistency).

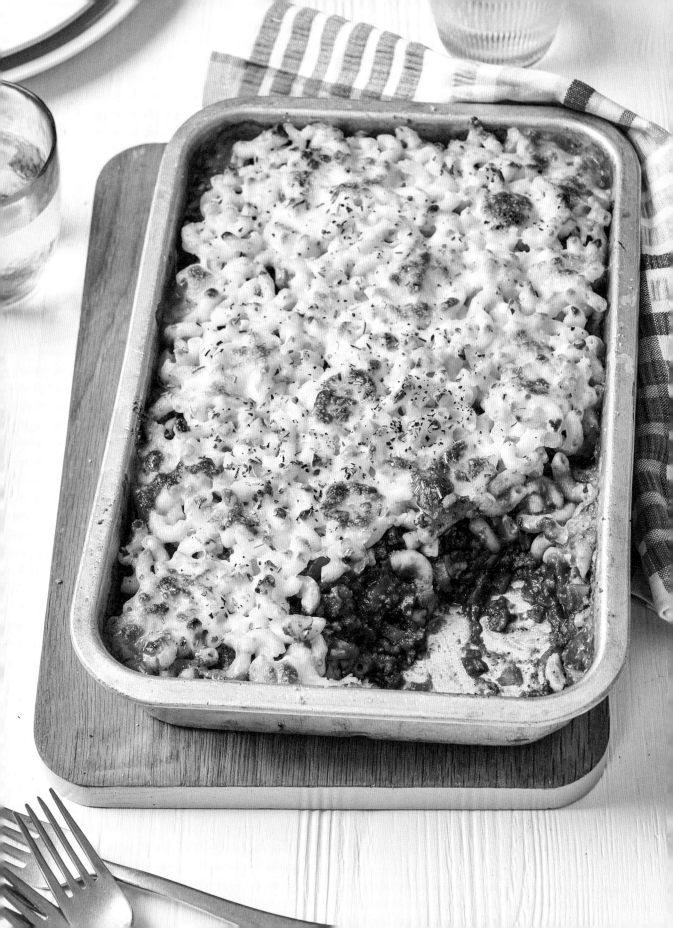

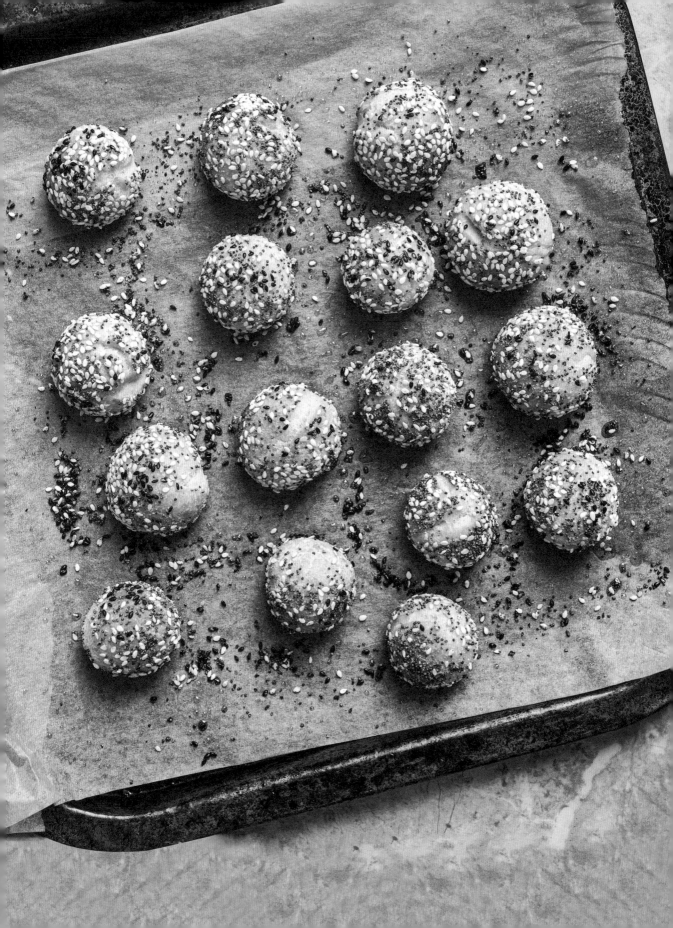

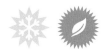

EVERYTHING SEASONED DOUGH BALLS

MAKES 16
PREP TIME: 5 MINUTES
COOK TIME: 15 MINUTES

150g (5½oz) self-raising flour, plus more to dust, if needed

pinch of salt

150g (5½oz) fat-free Greek yogurt

3 tablespoons Everything Seasoning (see page 224)

spray oil, or low-calorie cooking spray

Dough balls are one of my daughters' favourite teatime treats, so it's handy to have this easy and healthy version which can be whipped up in just 20 minutes. The mix of flavours in Everything Seasoning really complements these perfectly, but you can also keep them plain and stick to a simple garlic butter glaze.

1   Preheat the oven to 210°C/190°C fan (410°F), Gas Mark 6½.

2   Put the flour and a pinch of salt in a large mixing bowl, then add the yogurt. Please note that yogurt can really vary in consistency, so if yours seems quite watery, you may need a little less than the recipe states, or if it's very thick you may need a little more.

3   Use a table knife or spoon to bring the dough together as much as you can, then go in with your hands to press and form it into a ball of dough. I get roughly equal-sized balls out of this by splitting the ball of dough in half, then splitting each half in half and repeating until I have 16 pieces.

4   Put the 3 tablespoons of everything seasoning on to a side plate.

5   Roll each piece of dough between your palms to form a smooth ball (dust it with a little extra flour if it's too sticky), then roll it through the everything seasoning and place on a large baking tray. Repeat with all 16 balls. Spray with some oil, or low-calorie cooking spray.

6   Place on the middle shelf of the oven and bake for 15 minutes. Have a little look after 12 minutes just to make sure that they aren't browning too much: they should be golden brown but not dark brown. Serve hot from the oven.

PER DOUGH BALL
CALORIES 50
FAT 1.2G
SAT FAT 0.2G
CARBS 7.3G
SUGARS 0.5G
FIBRE 0.6G
PROTEIN 2.2G
SALT 0.15G

Note

To make a garlicky butter dip, put 2 tablespoons (30g / 1oz) butter in a small, microwave-safe bowl. Crush in 2 garlic cloves, then microwave for 20–30 seconds, until the butter is melted, stirring in the garlic. Once the plain dough balls are cooked, use a pastry brush to brush each one with the garlic butter while still warm.

- ✓ EAT~UP SUNDAY CURRY
- ✓ MOROCCAN~STYLE ROAST CHICKEN WITH SWEET POTATO COUSCOUS
- ✓ CHEAT'S CASSOULET
- ✓ SLOW~COOKER GINGER BEER HAM
- ✓ PORK, APPLE, SAGE AND LEEK CASSEROLE
- ✓ SLOW~COOKER MUSHROOM BOURGUIGNON
- ✓ SLOW~COOKER SCOTTISH STOVIES WITH BRISKET
- ✓ POT~ROAST BEEF WITH RED WINE GRAVY
- ✓ ULTIMATE BOLOGNESE SAUCE
- ✓ BEEF AND STOUT HOTPOT

7

Staples Sunday

EAT-UP SUNDAY CURRY

SERVES 6
PREP TIME: 10 MINUTES
COOK TIME: 1 HOUR

spray oil

2 onions, chopped

3 skinless chicken breasts

4 garlic cloves, crushed

5cm (2 inch) piece of fresh root ginger, peeled and finely grated or finely chopped

2 tablespoons mild tandoori curry powder

400g (14oz) can of chopped tomatoes

400g (14oz) can of light coconut milk

600g (1lb 5oz) potatoes, cut into bite-sized chunks

150g (5½oz) dried red lentils

400g (14oz) can of chickpeas, drained

1 tablespoon mango chutney

1 teaspoon coarse ground salt

TO SERVE

coriander, basil, parsley or mint leaves

chilli sauce, such as sriracha

This is designed as a super-easy option for a family meal that the kids can enjoy as much as the grown-ups. Rather than multiple spices, I've just used a supermarket mild tandoori spice mix, so there's no chilli heat in this, just flavour, and it's a great introduction to curry for younger children. There are no 'suspicious' ingredients, just simple chicken, potatoes, chickpeas and red lentils, all ingredients that work well for fussier eaters. A mild, creamy coconut milk-and-tomato sauce makes this a winner in my household, as my fussy eaters even ask for seconds! You can serve this with rice if you wish, but there's enough body and filling-power to mean it's also perfect just on its own in a bowl, or with some naan or pitta bread. Hopefully you'll have leftovers for easy lunches during the week, or to pop into the freezer.

1 Spray a large flameproof casserole pot with oil and place over a medium heat. Fry the onions and whole chicken breasts for 8 minutes, stirring every now and again.

2 Add the garlic, ginger and curry powder and stir-fry for another minute.

3 Pour in the chopped tomatoes, then fill the can with water and add that to the pan too. Add the coconut milk, potatoes, red lentils, chickpeas, mango chutney and salt, give everything a good stir and leave to simmer for 45 minutes, stirring occasionally to prevent anything sticking to the bottom of the pan.

4 After 45 minutes, remove the chicken breasts from the pan to a chopping board and thinly slice, then return the meat to the curry and stir in.

5 Serve scattered with the herbs of your choice. I always add a drizzle of chilli sauce to my portion.

PER SERVING
CALORIES 415
FAT 8G
SAT FAT 4.6G
CARBS 48G
SUGARS 11G
FIBRE 7.7G
PROTEIN 33G
SALT 1.2G

Note

There's a lot of potential to customize this curry to taste, or to make it vegetarian. For a vegetarian version, leave out the chicken in step 1, and in step 3 add chopped-up sweet potatoes, pumpkin or squash, cauliflower, broccoli, carrots or peppers. You could also add spinach, kale, green beans or baby corn towards the end of the cooking time.

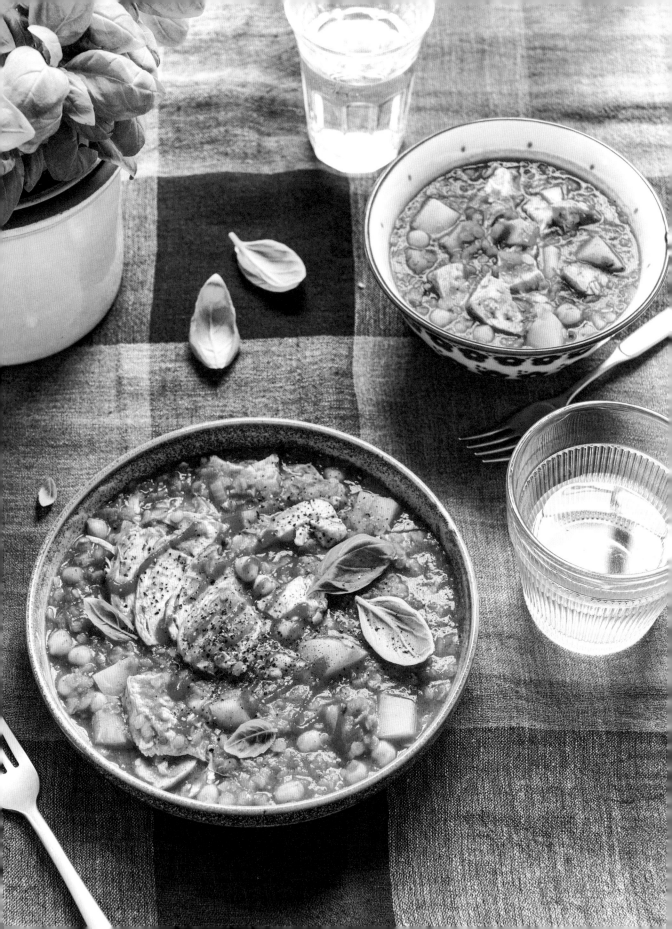

MOROCCAN-STYLE ROAST CHICKEN WITH SWEET POTATO COUSCOUS

SERVES 6
PREP TIME: 20 MINUTES
COOK TIME: 1½ HOURS

2 tablespoons fat-free Greek yogurt

1 tablespoon honey

1 teaspoon ground cumin

1 teaspoon garlic granules

½ teaspoon smoked paprika, plus a little more for sprinkling

½ teaspoon ground cinnamon

½ teaspoon coarse ground salt

2 lemons, 1 zested then halved, 1 juiced

1 whole chicken (about 1.5kg / 3lb 5oz)

3 red onions, thinly sliced

about 500g (1lb 5oz) sweet potato, peeled and chopped into 5mm (¼ inch) cubes

400g (14oz) can of chickpeas, drained and rinsed

spray oil, or low-calorie cooking spray

250g (9oz) wholewheat couscous

300ml (½ pint) boiling-hot vegetable stock

large handful of mint leaves, finely chopped

salt and pepper

I love to mix up a Sunday roast by adding different spices or flavourings to the chicken, then theming the accompaniments around that. I find fat-free Greek yogurt a great alternative to butter as a vehicle to help the flavours absorb into the chicken. The Moroccan-inspired flavours used here are fragrant but not spicy, so they're ideal for a family meal. I make the most of having the oven on for the chicken by roasting some vegetables to make a tasty couscous, then serve this with whatever green vegetables I have in.

1   Preheat the oven to 200°C/180°C fan (400°F), Gas Mark 6.

2   In a small bowl, mix the yogurt, honey, cumin, garlic granules, smoked paprika, ground cinnamon, salt and lemon zest to combine thoroughly.

3   Place the chicken in a roasting tin. Slide your fingers under the skin around the breast meat to loosen it enough to be able to spread half the spiced yogurt underneath the skin and over both breasts (I use a teaspoon to get it under the skin and start to spread, then use my fingers to spread it around as much as I can). Rub the remaining spiced yogurt over the whole outside of the chicken and place the lemon halves inside it.

4   Cover the roasting tin with a large piece of foil, 'tenting' it over the top of the chicken so that it doesn't touch it and sealing it as firmly as you can around the edges. If your foil is too narrow, use 2 pieces to achieve the same effect, making sure the sheets aren't resting on top of the chicken skin. Place the chicken in the oven and set the timer for 1 hour.

5   After 1 hour, place the onions, sweet potato cubes and chickpeas into another large roasting tin and spray them with oil, or low-calorie cooking spray, season with salt and pepper and give them a good mix. Remove the chicken from the oven and take off the foil (save this for later), then pop the chicken and the vegetables and chickpeas back into the oven to roast, setting a timer for 20 minutes.

6   Give the vegetables and chickpeas a good stir and return them to the oven, then remove the chicken from the oven. Check it's cooked by inserting a sharp knife into the thickest part of the leg and checking the juices run clear (or use a meat thermometer; it should measure an internal temperature of 75°C / 167°F). Cover the chicken with the reserved foil and leave it to rest while you prepare the couscous.

7   Pour the couscous into a medium-sized heatproof bowl and pour in the boiling-hot stock. Cover with a plate or foil and leave for 10 minutes. Remove the roast vegetables and chickpeas from the oven and set to the side until the couscous is ready.

8   Use a fork to fluff up the couscous, then put it in a large bowl with the chopped mint, roasted vegetables and chickpeas and the juice of the remaining lemon. Mix together, then cover the bowl with a plate or foil while you carve the chicken.

9   Serve the chicken with the warm couscous.

PER SERVING
CALORIES 549
FAT 24G
SAT FAT 6.6G
CARBS 41G
SUGARS 26G
FIBRE 5G
PROTEIN 38G
SALT 0.92G

Note

You may have to adjust your cooking times for the chicken depending on its size. Many supermarkets now label the packaging with the correct cooking time.

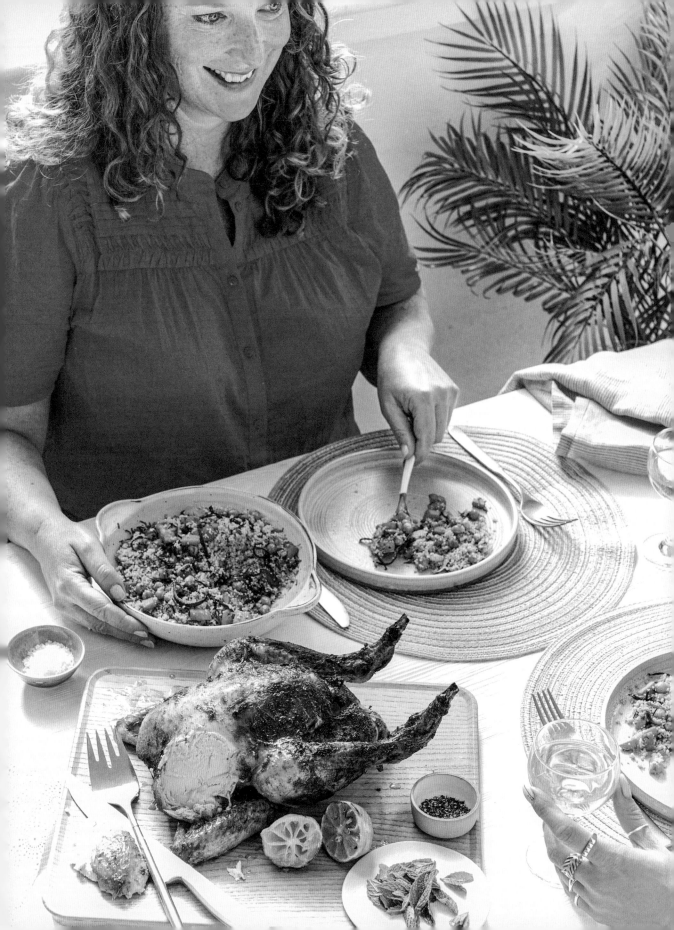

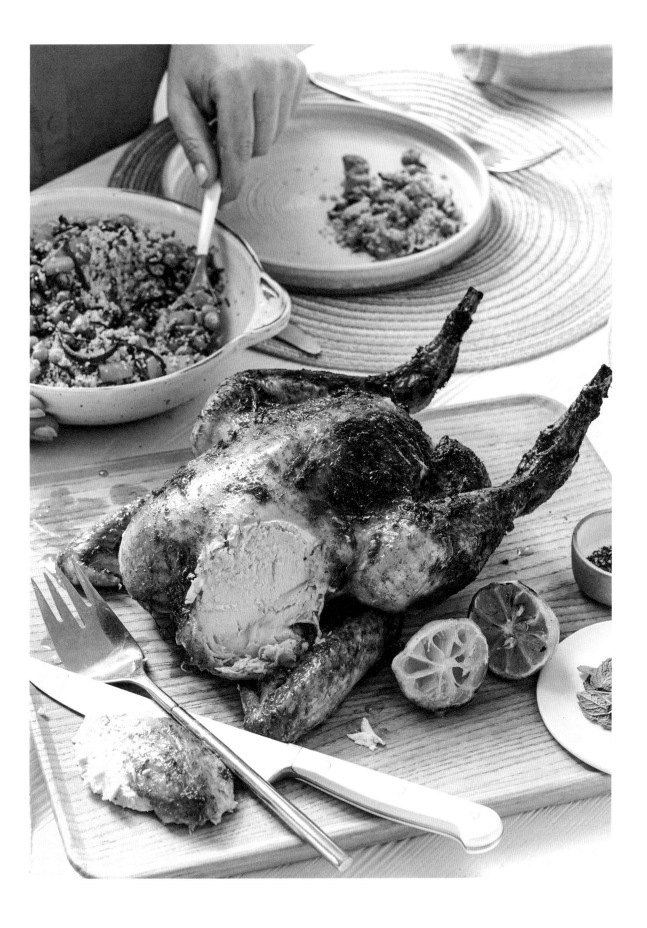

CHEAT'S CASSOULET

SERVES 6
PREP TIME: 20 MINUTES
COOK TIME: 1¼ HOURS

spray oil

4 reduced-fat pork sausages, each chopped into 6

1 smoked gammon steak, thinly sliced

3 skinless chicken thigh fillets, thinly sliced

1 large onion, sliced

6 garlic cloves, chopped

1 carrot, chopped

2 celery stalks, finely sliced

½ teaspoon fennel seeds

800ml (1 pint 8fl oz) hot chicken stock

2 tablespoons red wine vinegar

2 tablespoons tomato purée

2 teaspoons dried rosemary

2 teaspoons smoked paprika

2 x 400g (14oz) cans of haricot beans, drained

400g (14oz) can of butter beans, drained

large handful of parsley leaves, finely chopped

50g (1¾oz) panko breadcrumbs

salt and pepper

My mum often used to make cassoulet for big family gatherings. It's a traditional French bean-and-meat stew slow-cooked with plenty of garlic and herbs, and has many regional variations. In an ideal world, we would all slow-cook our cassoulet and have the budget to add traditional ingredients such as duck and Toulouse sausages. I think it's a real shame for us home cooks to miss out on this delicious meal, or be put off making it, because we don't have those meats. So although my version is not authentic by any means (especially the low-fat aspect!) it is still hearty comfort food, great for feeding a crowd and, if you want to add duck and special sausage, then please do. This really is great mopped up with some fresh bread, and seasonal green vegetables are another wonderful accompaniment.

1 Spray a large casserole dish, which has a lid, with oil and place over a medium heat. Add the sausages, gammon and chicken and stir-fry for 10 minutes.

2 Add the onion, garlic, carrot and celery and stir-fry for another 5 minutes.

3 Stir through the fennel seeds, then pour in the hot chicken stock. Add the red wine vinegar, tomato purée, rosemary, smoked paprika and all the beans, then season with salt and pepper.

4 Stir through the parsley, then simmer with the lid off for 20 minutes.

5 Reduce the heat slightly and simmer, lid on, for another 30 minutes, stirring every now and again. Preheat the grill to high.

6 Turn off the heat, give the cassoulet a final stir, then evenly scatter the panko breadcrumbs over the top. Spray all over with a little oil, season with a few grinds of salt and pepper, then place under the hot grill for 5 minutes, until the breadcrumbs have turned a golden brown colour.

7 Serve the casserole dish at the table and let everyone help themselves.

PER SERVING
CALORIES 401
FAT 7.3G
SAT FAT 2.2G
CARBS 37G
SUGARS 6.3G
FIBRE 9.9G
PROTEIN 40G
SALT 2.6G

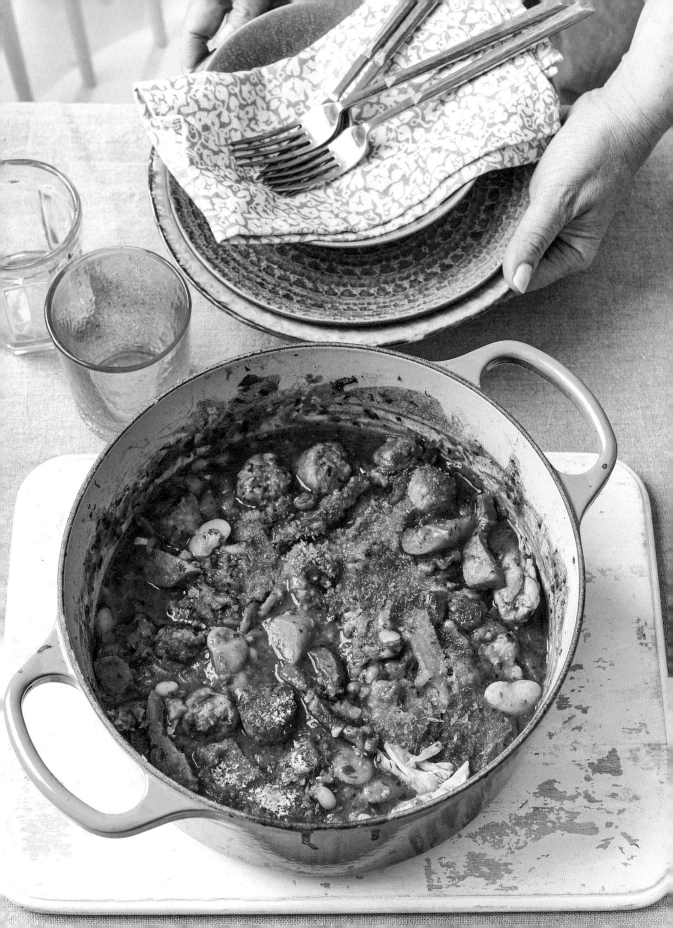

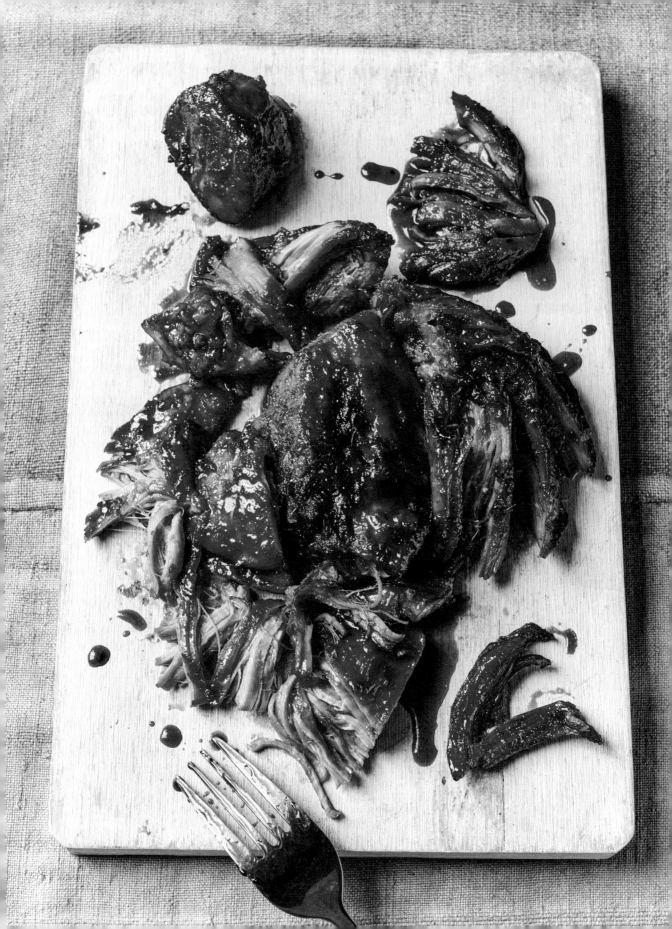

SLOW-COOKER GINGER BEER HAM

SERVES 6
PREP TIME: 5 MINUTES
COOK TIME: HIGH 4–5 HOURS,
LOW 7–8 HOURS,
PLUS 12–15 MINUTES TO GLAZE
(OPTIONAL)

2cm (¾ inch) fresh root ginger, cut into thin slices
1kg (2lb 4oz) unsmoked gammon joint
750ml (1 pint 6fl oz) ginger beer

FOR THE GLAZE (OPTIONAL)
2 tablespoons honey
1 tablespoon dark soy sauce
1 teaspoon ginger purée

The slow-cooker is a great way to cook ham: it saves having to keep an eye on it on the hob and it allows plenty of time for flavour to infuse. I love it with a subtle hint of ginger from ginger beer, it just gives a little something extra, especially if you add the oven-glazing step right at the end of the cooking time. I don't think you can beat ham served with chips, beans and a fried egg, but this is also great in sandwiches, as part of a lunch of cold cuts, cheese and salad, or cut up and added to soup, pasta or quiche. I use ready-made ginger purée for the glaze here, as it gives better coverage than freshly grated and doesn't leave any bits sticking on the ham.

1   Place the ginger slices at the bottom of the slow-cooker pot, put the gammon in and pour over the ginger beer. If the ham isn't fully immersed, just top up with water so it's covered. Cook on high for 4–5 hours, or on low for 7–8 hours.

2   If you want to glaze the ham, preheat the oven to 220°C/200°C fan (425°F), Gas Mark 7 towards the end of its cooking time in the slow-cooker.

3   Lift the ham out of the slow-cooker on to a carving dish, snip away any string, then use a sharp knife to slice away the thick layer of fat from the top of the ham (discard this), leaving just a very thin layer of fat. Now use the sharp knife to score across the top of the ham in a criss-cross pattern.

4   Line a baking tin with foil, then put the ham in, fat-side up.

5   Mix the glaze ingredients in a small bowl, then spoon this over the ham, making sure it fully covers the top.

6   Put the tray into the oven and bake for 12–15 minutes until the top of the ham is a glistening, golden brown.

7   Thinly slice the ham to serve (or see recipe introduction).

PER SERVING
CALORIES 344
FAT 10G
SAT FAT 3.8G
CARBS 19G
SUGARS 15G
FIBRE 1G
PROTEIN 43G
SALT 3.3G

Note

Want to make this without a slow-cooker? First of all, work out the cooking time. You need to calculate 20 minutes per 450g (1lb), plus an extra 20 minutes (so a 1kg / 2lb 4oz gammon will need 64 minutes). Boil the ham in the ginger and ginger beer for half the cooking time (32 minutes in this case), then roast it for the remainder of the cooking time in an oven preheated to 200°C/180°C fan (400°F), Gas Mark 6. For the last 15 minutes of cooking time, remove the top layer of fat, following steps 2–3 in the recipe above, glaze, then return to the oven for the final 15 minutes.

PORK, APPLE, SAGE & LEEK CASSEROLE

SERVES 4
PREP TIME: 15 MINUTES
COOK TIME: 30 MINUTES

spray oil

2 onions, finely chopped

2 celery stalks, finely chopped

2 leeks, trimmed, cleaned and sliced into 1cm (½ inch) pieces

500g (1lb 2oz) lean minced pork (less than 5 per cent fat)

1 tablespoon cornflour

1 tablespoon dried sage

2 teaspoons mustard powder

2 tablespoons cider vinegar

800ml (1 pint 8fl oz) hot chicken stock

2 apples, cored and chopped

650g (1lb 7oz) potatoes, chopped

salt and pepper

A delicious, hearty all-in-one casserole that is great for the whole family. Pork, leek, apple and sage make such a gorgeous flavour combination, while using minced pork here not only makes the meat go further, but is cheaper, quicker to cook and also easy for younger kids to eat.

1 Spray a large casserole with oil and place over a medium-high heat. Fry the onions, celery and leeks for 5 minutes.

2 Add the pork and cornflour and stir-fry for 5 more minutes, breaking up clumps in the minced meat with your spoon.

3 Stir the sage, mustard powder, cider vinegar and seasoning into the pan, then pour in the chicken stock. Add the apples and potatoes, stir well and simmer for 20 minutes, until the potatoes are tender.

4 Divide between 4 bowls and serve.

PER SERVING
CALORIES 455
FAT 8G
SAT FAT 2.7G
CARBS 55G
SUGARS 19G
FIBRE 8.1G
PROTEIN 37G
SALT 1.8G

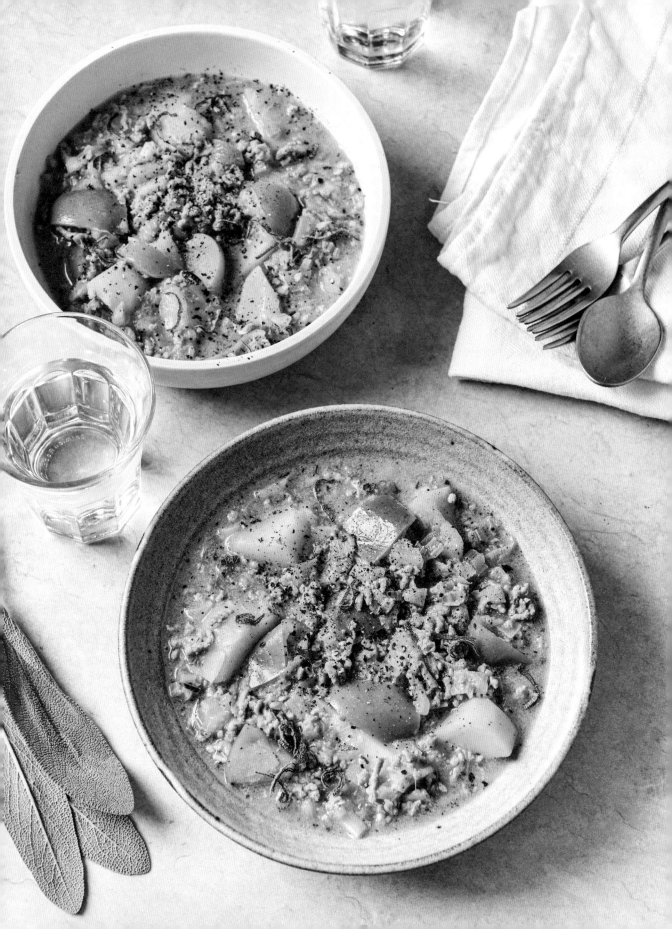

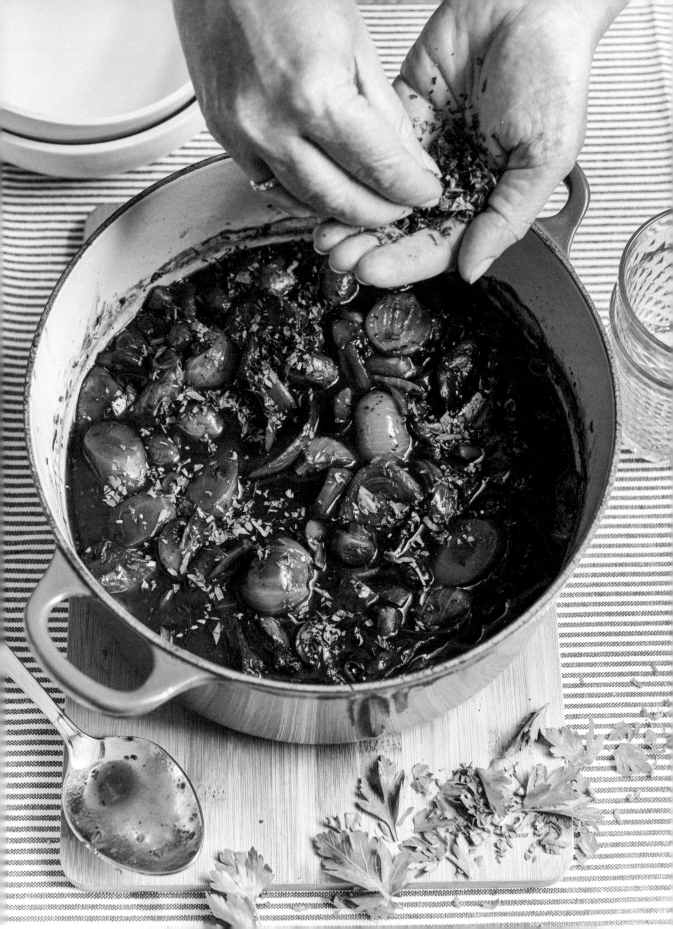

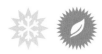

SLOW-COOKER MUSHROOM BOURGUIGNON

SERVES 4
PREP TIME: 20 MINUTES
COOK TIME: 5 HOURS,
PLUS 10 MINUTES

25g (1oz) dried porcini mushrooms

1 tablespoon (15g / ½oz) butter

350g (12oz) shallots (see note), halved

2 large carrots, sliced

3 garlic cloves, crushed

2 tablespoons tomato purée

2 tablespoons cornflour

200ml (7fl oz) red wine

1 teaspoon Marmite, or other yeast extract

1 teaspoon dried rosemary

1 teaspoon dried thyme

1 teaspoon dried basil

1 teaspoon coarse ground salt

½ teaspoon freshly ground black pepper

250g (9oz) chestnut mushrooms, quartered

250g (9oz) large flat/portobello mushrooms, halved and thickly sliced

200g (7oz) baby button mushrooms

450ml (16fl oz) hot vegetable stock

chopped parsley leaves, to serve

I'm delighted to say that this captures the delicious, deep flavours of beef bourguignon, but makes mushrooms the star of the dish for a vegetarian-friendly meal. I like to serve this with mashed potatoes, boulangère potatoes (see page 219) or rice, with asparagus or other seasonal green vegetables.

1 Place the porcini mushrooms in a small bowl and pour over enough freshly boiled water just to cover.

2 Melt the butter in a sauté pan over a medium-high heat and fry the shallots for 5 minutes. Stir through the carrots and garlic and fry for another couple of minutes, then transfer them to the slow-cooker pot.

3 In a small bowl, mix the tomato purée and cornflour to form a smooth paste. Spoon into the sauté pan, set over a low heat, then slowly stir in the red wine a bit at a time to form a smooth, lump-free sauce.

4 Add the Marmite or yeast extract, dried herbs, salt and pepper, stir well, bring to the boil, then turn off the heat.

5 Add all the mushrooms to the slow-cooker pot, including the porcini mushrooms and the water they have been soaking in. Pour in the red wine sauce, using a spatula to make sure you've got it all out of the pan and into the pot. Pour over the vegetable stock.

6 Cook on low for 5 hours. If you are around to stir it halfway through, then do, but this is not imperative.

Note

PER SERVING
CALORIES 213
FAT 4.7G
SAT FAT 2.4G
CARBS 22G
SUGARS 9.8G
FIBRE 8.8G
PROTEIN 7.6G
SALT 1.6G

> Want to make this without a slow-cooker? Use a large casserole pot to start frying the shallots, then follow the recipe up to the end of step 4. Using some spray oil, fry the mushrooms separately (you may need to do this in batches so as not to overcrowd the pan), then add the fried mushrooms, porcini mushrooms and stock to the pot and simmer for 25 minutes, stirring every now and again.

> To make shallots easier to peel, soak them in freshly boiled water for 10 minutes, then drain, cut away the root and peel them. If you don't have time to prepare shallots, simply replace them in this recipe with 1 large chopped regular onion.

SLOW-COOKER SCOTTISH STOVIES WITH **BRISKET**

SERVES 4
PREP TIME: 15 MINUTES
COOK TIME: HIGH 6–8 HOURS,
LOW 10–12 HOURS,
PLUS 10 MINUTES

1 tablespoon butter

2 large onions, finely sliced

900g (2lb) Maris Piper potatoes, peeled and sliced into 1cm (½ inch) slices

1 tablespoon cornflour

500ml (18fl oz) hot beef stock

1 tablespoon Worcestershire sauce, or Henderson's relish

1 tablespoon brown sauce

500g (1lb 2oz) beef brisket, fat trimmed away

3–4 carrots (total weight about 200g / 7oz), peeled and sliced

salt and pepper

Scots are very passionate about the right way to cook stovies... there are many 'right ways' and family recipes with all sorts of variations. If you haven't heard of stovies, it is a slow-cooked dish containing potatoes, onion and meat. The meat used is generally the leftovers from a roast dinner, usually beef or lamb, or sometimes sausage or corned beef. I make mine with a beef brisket joint in the slow cooker. As I don't use the traditional beef dripping for flavour, I make a couple of additions which may not be authentic but do add lovely flavour to this ultimate comfort food. This is a meal in one, but can be eaten with Scottish Oatcakes (see page 222) and pickled beetroot.

1   Melt the butter in a saucepan, add the onions and start them frying (they need to fry for about 10 minutes until soft and golden) while you peel and slice the potatoes.

2   Put the cornflour in a small bowl or ramekin, add about 3 tablespoons cold water and stir to make a smooth paste.

3   Make up the beef stock in a jug and stir in the Worcestershire sauce or Henderson's relish, the brown sauce and the cornflour mixture.

4   Arrange a layer of potatoes in the bottom of the slow-cooker pot. Place the beef brisket on top, season it with salt and pepper, then add the rest of the potato, the fried onions and the carrots all around it.

5   Pour over the gravy, pop the lid on and cook on high for 6–8 hours, or low for 10–12 hours. At the end of the cooking time, you should be able to easily shred the meat.

PER SERVING
CALORIES 504
FAT 12G
SAT FAT 5.3G
CARBS 61G
SUGARS 15G
FIBRE 9.8G
PROTEIN 34G
SALT 1.5G

> Beef briskets often come in a larger size – 800g–1kg (1lb 12oz–2lb 4oz) – so if you have one of those, simply cut it in half and freeze half for another meal.

> Want to make this without a slow-cooker? Cook in a casserole with a tight-fitting lid at 170°C/150°C fan (340°CF), Gas Mark 3½ for 4 hours. Check on it about halfway through cooking, turn the meat over and top up with a little hot stock if it looks like it might be drying out.

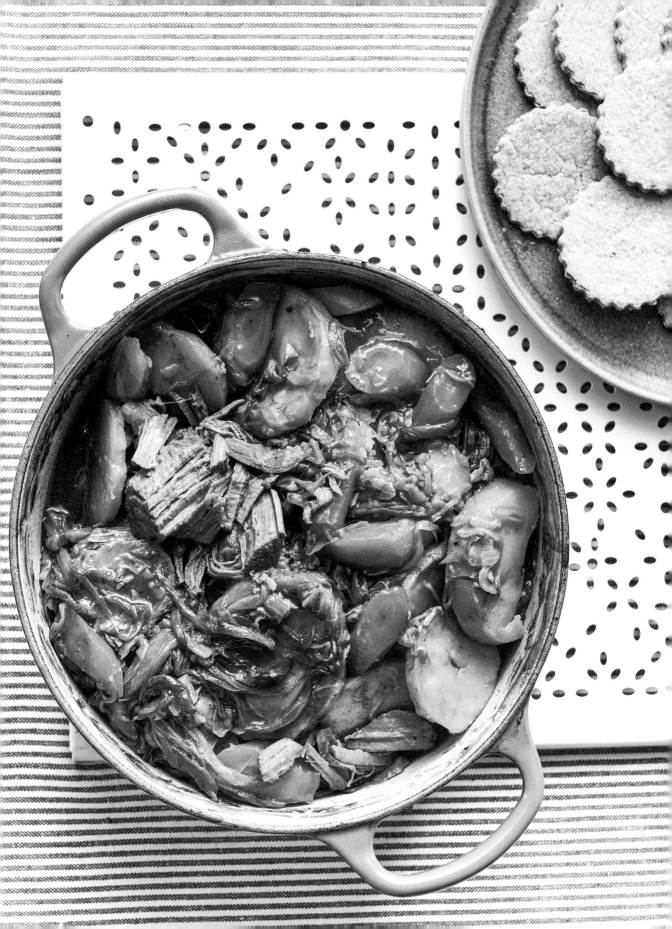

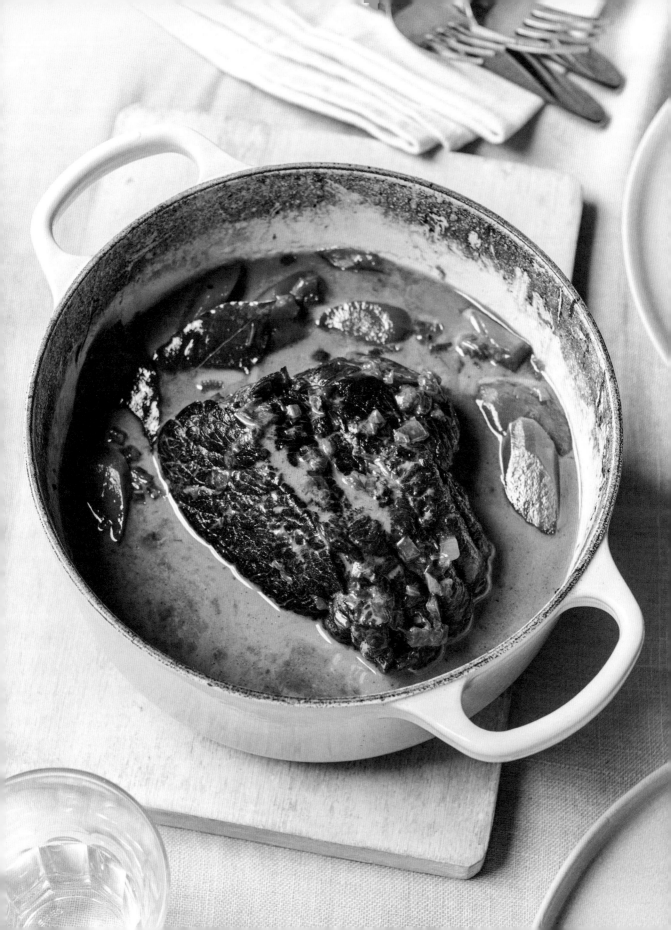

POT-ROAST BEEF WITH RED WINE GRAVY

SERVES 4
PREP TIME: 10 MINUTES
COOK TIME: 2¼ HOURS

spray oil

1kg (2lb 4oz) topside or silverside of beef

1 onion, chopped

4 carrots, sliced

2 celery stalks, finely chopped

2 garlic cloves, crushed

200ml (7fl oz) red wine

2 teaspoons blackcurrant jam, or redcurrant jelly

600ml (20fl oz) hot beef stock

2 bay leaves

salt and pepper

This is a failsafe way to make tender roast beef with rich gravy. And it's not only easy to do, but also very little work. Topside and silverside are both readily available lean cuts of beef, but roasting them in the usual fashion can result in a disappointingly chewy result. By cooking the beef already in its own gravy, not only is it beautifully tender to slice, but you also don't have to make a separate gravy. Serve this with your favourite potatoes (mash or roast) and vegetables; depending on what you serve alongside, it could easily stretch to feed six.

1   Preheat the oven to 180°C/160°C fan (350°F), Gas Mark 4.

2   Spray a frying pan with a little oil and set it over a medium heat. Place the beef in the pan and spray it all over with oil. Fry for about 5 minutes, turning it over every minute or so to brown and sear it on all sides.

3   Remove the beef from the frying pan and place it in a large ovenproof casserole pot which has a lid. Season with salt and pepper.

4   Put the onion, carrots and celery into the frying pan and fry for about 5 minutes, then stir in the garlic and fry for 1 more minute. Pour in the red wine, bring to the boil and simmer for 1 minute, then stir in the jam or jelly. Transfer this mixture to the casserole pot with the beef, then pour in the beef stock and add the bay leaves.

5   Pop the lid on the pot and transfer it to the middle shelf of the oven. Cook for 2 hours, turning the beef over halfway through cooking.

6   When you remove the pot from the oven, lift the beef out on to a chopping board or carving tray. Carve the beef into thin slices.

7   Transfer the gravy to a large jug and serve alongside the beef.

PER SERVING
CALORIES 443
FAT 12G
SAT FAT 4.2G
CARBS 10G
SUGARS 8.3G
FIBRE 3.9G
PROTEIN 62G
SALT 1.6G

Note

This gravy isn't thick, which is how I like it. If you prefer a thick gravy, mix 1 tablespoon cornflour with a little cold water in a cup and stir until smooth. Once you have removed the beef from the gravy, place the pot of gravy back over a medium heat and add the cornflour mix. Bring it to a simmer and cook for about 5 minutes, stirring, until the gravy thickens.

ULTIMATE BOLOGNESE SAUCE

SERVES 6
PREP TIME: 10 MINUTES
COOK TIME: 1 HOUR 5 MINUTES

2 onions, halved

2 celery stalks, roughly chopped

3 medium carrots, roughly chopped

4 garlic cloves

1 tablespoon olive oil

500g (1lb 2oz) lean minced beef (less than 5 per cent fat)

200g (7oz) lean minced pork (less than 5 per cent fat)

2 x 400g (14oz) cans of chopped tomatoes

4 tablespoons tomato purée

1 beef stock cube or pot (cube crumbled, or stock pot dissolved in a little boiling water)

1 tablespoon dark soy sauce

1 tablespoon honey

1 teaspoon dried oregano

1 teaspoon dried basil

1 teaspoon coarse ground salt

¼ teaspoon freshly ground black pepper

200ml (7fl oz) semi-skimmed milk

Spaghetti Bolognese is a family favourite for a reason. It's one of my most-loved go-to Sunday meals as it doesn't take as much work or time as a roast, and you can have it ready in advance, but everyone digs in and enjoys it. I was always very fussy about textures as a child, so my mum used to purée Bolognese sauce for me so there weren't any lumpy bits. This version is a nod to that habit, as I blend the onion, carrots, celery and tomatoes both for speed (saves a lot of chopping!) but also to avoid fussiness from the kids. I've used a mixture of pork and beef, but if you don't eat pork you can just use beef. Serve with your favourite pasta and green veg and freeze any leftovers for an easy meal another day.

1   Place the onions, celery, carrots and garlic in a food processor and whizz until very finely chopped.

2   Put the olive oil in a large sauté pan or flameproof casserole dish, and place over a medium heat. Use a spatula to scrape in the vegetables from the processor bowl. Fry them for 10 minutes, stirring every now and again.

3   Push the vegetables over to one side of the pan and place the minced meat on the other side, breaking up the clumps with a wooden spoon and stir-frying until it is mainly browned (about 5 minutes).

4   Add the chopped tomatoes to the food processor bowl and whizz these up until they are smooth and lump-free. Pour the chopped tomatoes into the pan, then add the tomato purée, beef stock, soy sauce, honey, oregano, basil and salt and pepper. Mix well, then leave to simmer gently for 40 minutes, stirring every now and again.

5   Pour the milk into the sauce, stir it in, then leave it to simmer for a final 10 minutes before serving.

PER SERVING
CALORIES 333
FAT 9.1G
SAT FAT 3.1G
CARBS 21G
SUGARS 19G
FIBRE 5.8G
PROTEIN 37G
SALT 2G

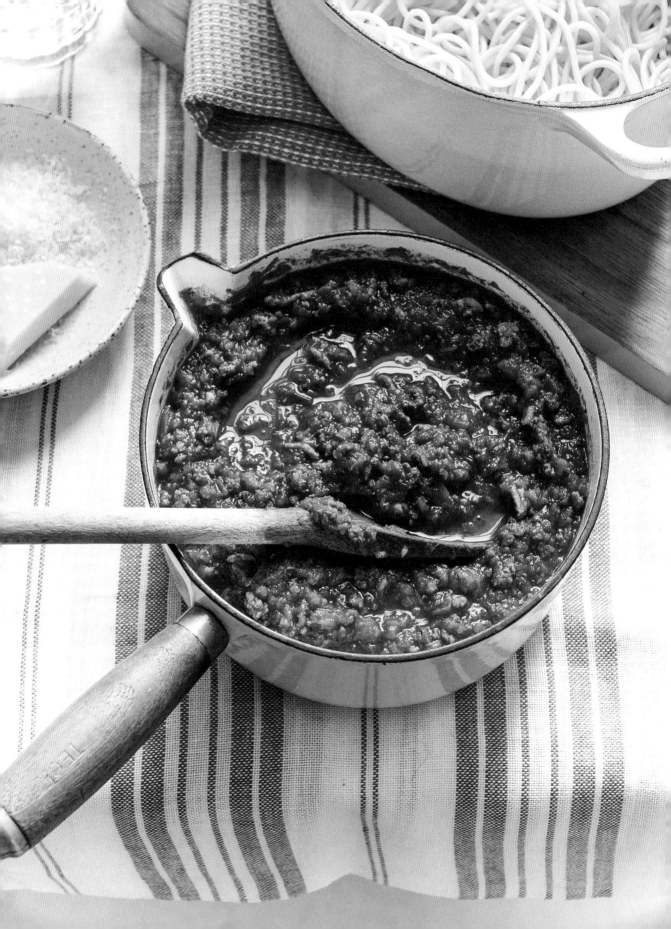

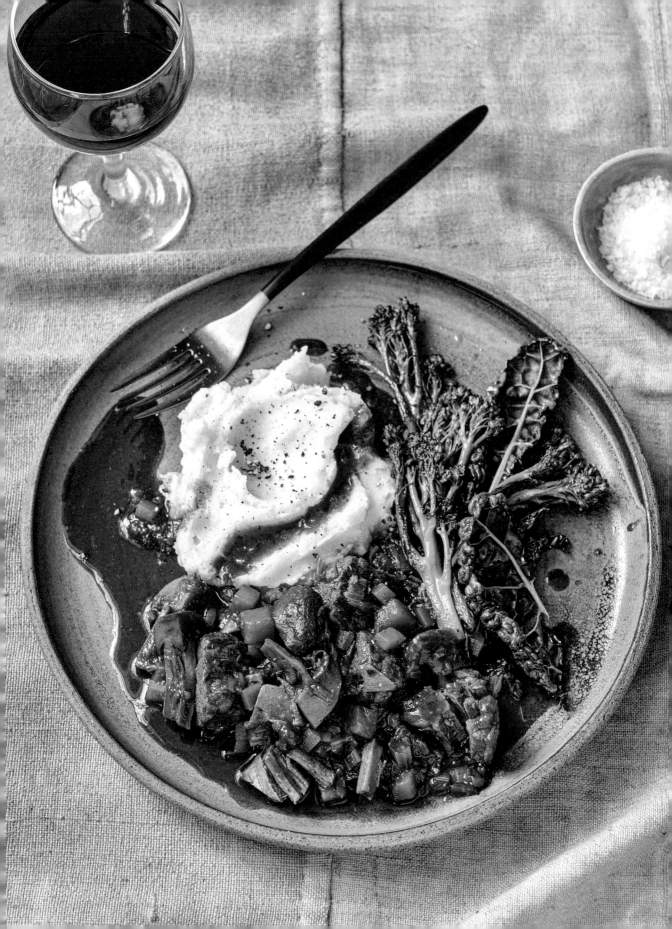

BEEF & STOUT HOTPOT

SERVES 6
PREP TIME: 20 MINUTES
COOK TIME: 3 HOURS 10 MINUTES

spray oil

800g (1lb 12oz) lean beef brisket, all fat trimmed away, cut into chunks

2 onions, chopped

2 celery stalks, finely chopped

2 garlic cloves, crushed

2 tablespoons tomato purée

1 tablespoon cornflour

500ml (18fl oz) stout

400ml (14fl oz) hot beef stock

1 bay leaf

½ teaspoon dried rosemary

½ teaspoon dried thyme

2 carrots, finely chopped

1 small swede (about 150g / 5½oz), peeled and finely chopped

250g (9oz) chestnut mushrooms, quartered

1 tablespoon dark soy sauce

salt and pepper

Beef and stout (a dark, full-bodied ale such as Guinness) stew must be one of the best comfort food meals out there and it makes a great family meal. I use beef brisket to make mine, as it's a great lean cut which slow-cooks perfectly. Serve with mashed potato, roast potatoes, carrot and swede mash, or with your favourite seasonal green vegetables.

1 Preheat the oven to 180°C/160°C fan (350°F), Gas Mark 4.

2 Spray a large casserole dish with oil, add the beef chunks, onions, celery and garlic and stir-fry for 5 minutes.

3 Add the tomato purée and cornflour, stir them into the other ingredients, then pour in the stout.

4 Pour in the beef stock and add the herbs, carrots, swede, mushrooms, soy sauce and salt and pepper. Stir well, cover with a lid and place in the oven for 3 hours, giving it a stir halfway through.

5 Serve, removing the bay leaf as you do so.

PER SERVING
CALORIES 296
FAT 9.2G
SAT FAT 3.5G
CARBS 15G
SUGARS 11G
FIBRE 4.1G
PROTEIN 31G
SALT 1.2G

Note

To make this in a slow-cooker, put the beef chunks in the slow-cooker pot and stir them together with the cornflour. Add all the other ingredients apart from the stout and stock, stir together, then pour in the liquid. Cook on high for 6–8 hours, or low for 10–12 hours.

- ✓ RHUBARB AND CUSTARD CAKE
- ✓ RUSTIC `PROFITEROLES` WITH CARAMELIZED BISCUIT TOPPING
- ✓ GOLDEN SYRUP LOAF CAKE
- ✓ WATERMELON FINGERS WITH HONEY LIME DIP
- ✓ GINGERBREAD TREACLE MUFFINS
- ✓ SCHOOL-STYLE CHOCOLATE CRACKNELL
- ✓ JUST-RIGHT FLAPJACKS
- ✓ BLUEBERRY SCONES
- ✓ SHREWSBURY BISCUITS

8

Something Sweet

RHUBARB & CUSTARD CAKE

MAKES 12 SLICES
PREP TIME: 10 MINUTES
COOK TIME: 55 MINUTES

200g (7oz) reduced-fat cream cheese

150g (5½oz) caster sugar

4 eggs, lightly beaten

1 teaspoon vanilla extract

200g (7oz) self-raising flour

30g (1oz) custard power

1 teaspoon baking powder

200g (7oz) canned rhubarb, drained

a few drops of pink food colouring (optional)

This is a dense and moist loaf cake with a custard-flavoured crumb and pops of juicy rhubarb marbled throughout. The aim here, as usual, is for a healthier bake: it's still cake, to be enjoyed in moderation, but by replacing butter or margarine with reduced-fat cream cheese and cutting down on sugar, it's a little bit less of a blow-out than regular cake. For comparison, 200g (7oz) butter contains around 1,488 calories, 200g (7oz) margarine has around 1,255 calories, but 200g (7oz) reduced-fat cream cheese contains around 294 calories.

1   Preheat the oven to 180°C/160°C fan (350°F), Gas Mark 4. Line a 900g (2lb) loaf tin with nonstick baking paper, or a loaf tin liner.

2   In a large bowl, combine the cream cheese and sugar, then mix in the eggs and vanilla extract. Add the flour, custard powder and baking powder to the bowl and use a wooden spoon to mix everything into a smooth batter.

3   Put the canned rhubarb in a smaller bowl and add a little pink food colouring until you have a pleasing raspberry-pink colour. (This step is not essential, but I think the cake looks so much nicer with the pink colour rippling through it.)

4   Pour one-third of the cake batter into the prepared tin, then spoon half the rhubarb over the top as evenly as you can to cover as much of the batter as possible. Add another one-third of the batter, then the remaining rhubarb in the same way as before. Finish by covering with the remaining batter.

5   Place on the middle shelf of the oven and bake for 55 minutes, by which time the cake should be fully cooked through. Test this by inserting a sharp knife or cocktail stick into the middle. If it comes out clean the cake is done, but if it's coated in batter the cake needs a little longer cooking (cover it with foil if you are worried about the top browning too much).

6   Allow the cake to cool a little before cutting into 12 equal slices. You can store the cake for up to 3 days in an airtight container or well-wrapped in foil. You can individually freeze the slices, too.

PER SLICE
CALORIES 176
FAT 3.9G
SAT FAT 1.8G
CARBS 29G
SUGARS 14G
FIBRE 0.8G
PROTEIN 5.7G
SALT 0.45G

Note

If you prefer, you can use jam or conserve rather than canned rhubarb as the fruit filling for this cake. Rhubarb conserve has a much sweeter flavour than canned rhubarb, while other flavours such as blackcurrant will also make a delicious cake. Just be aware that this will affect the calorie content of the cake. If you freeze any leftovers, once you have defrosted a slice, try warming it through in the microwave and serving it up with hot custard: delicious!

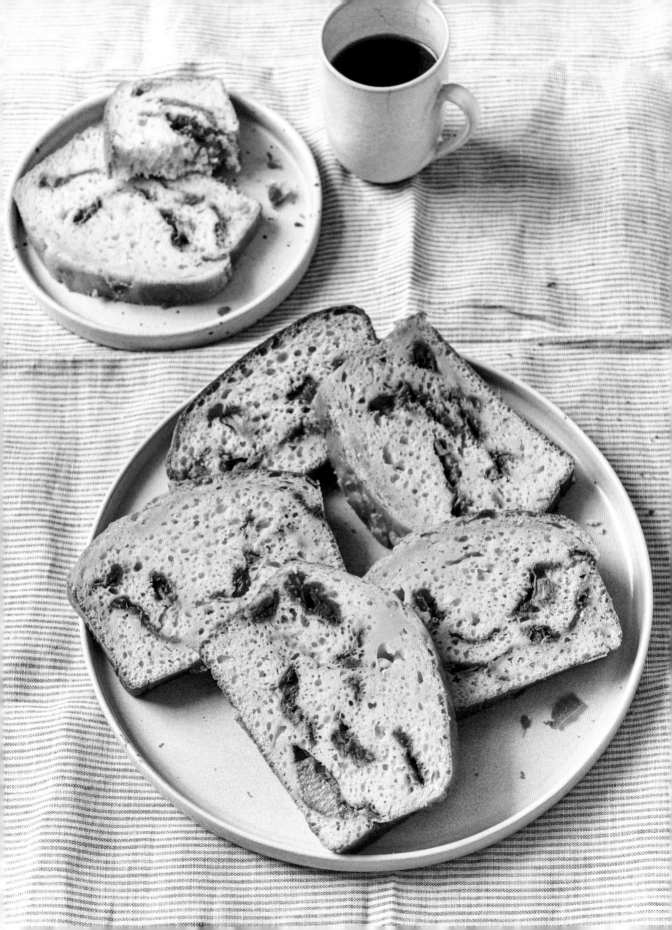

RUSTIC 'PROFITEROLES' WITH CARAMELIZED BISCUIT TOPPING

SERVES 12
PREP TIME: 20 MINUTES
COOK TIME: 20 MINUTES

low-calorie cooking spray

3 egg whites

2 teaspoons caster sugar

1 egg yolk

1 teaspoon vanilla extract

aerosol cream (about 60g / 2¼oz)

2 tablespoons Biscoff spread, or other caramelized biscuit spread

YOU WILL ALSO NEED

12 paper bun cases

12 hole bun tin or a 12 hole silicone bun tray

This is a complete cheat. It makes something resembling a profiterole, but would probably horrify any pastry chef! I absolutely love profiteroles, they are my favourite dessert, and these come close enough that – for me – they absolutely satisfy my cravings at less than half the calories of the real thing (using a standard supermarket profiterole for comparison). As a disclaimer, these aren't as perfectly formed as authentic profiteroles and, as they are filled with aerosol cream, they deflate in an hour or so. Although this means they aren't really something you can make in advance for a dinner party, inflating them with the cream is one of the most satisfying things to do and they still taste great even after they have deflated!

1   Preheat the oven to 180°C/160°C fan (350°F), Gas Mark 4. Line a 12-hole bun tin with 12 paper bun cases (if using a silicone tray then no need to use paper cases). Spray each bun case generously with low-calorie cooking spray: you need to ensure that the mixture doesn't stick to the cases.

2   In a large bowl, beat the egg whites until they form stiff peaks. I find doing this by hand takes about 3 minutes, but you can use an electric whisk if you have one. Add the sugar and whisk it into the egg whites.

3   In a small bowl or ramekin, beat up the egg yolk and add the vanilla extract, then use a metal spoon to fold this into the egg whites. Make sure it's completely combined, but be gentle and try not to knock too much air out of the egg whites.

4   Use a metal dessert spoon to scoop a generous dollop of mixture into each bun case. Try to keep the shape round, as much as possible. They should look like little snowballs, as they will bake in this shape and you want them to be as round as possible. They aren't going to be perfect, but a bit of care will allow you to get a uniform dollop in each case.

5   Put the baking tin on the middle shelf of the oven and bake for 20 minutes. Remove from the oven, remove the cases from the hot tin and place on a plate to cool more quickly. Leave to cool for at least 10 minutes. They are likely to deflate a bit, but that's fine.

6   Once they have cooled, very carefully peel away each paper bun case, trying not to tear the delicate 'pastry'. Use the handle of a teaspoon to make a small hole in the side of each and scoop it around gently inside to create a clear cavern for the cream.

7   Now insert the nozzle of the aerosol cream into the hole and fill the cream cavern. This is the satisfying bit: enjoy it as they puff up! Each profiterole will accommodate about 5g (1/8oz) of cream. Repeat this to fill all 12.

8   Place the Biscoff spread into a small bowl or ramekin and microwave for 1–1½ minutes to melt it. Drizzle this over the top of the profiteroles in a zig-zag pattern.

9   Allow 10 minutes for the Biscoff spread to set, then serve immediately, or store in the refrigerator. If you keep these in the refrigerator for more than 1 hour they will deflate slightly, but will still taste incredible.

PER PROFITEROLE
CALORIES 46
FAT 3.1G
SAT FAT 1.4G
CARBS 2.8G
SUGARS 2.3G
FIBRE 0G
PROTEIN 1.3G
SALT TRACE

Note

If you can get hold of chocolate aerosol cream, try a chocolate version of these by filling the buns with chocolate cream and topping them with chocolate spread, softened in the microwave.

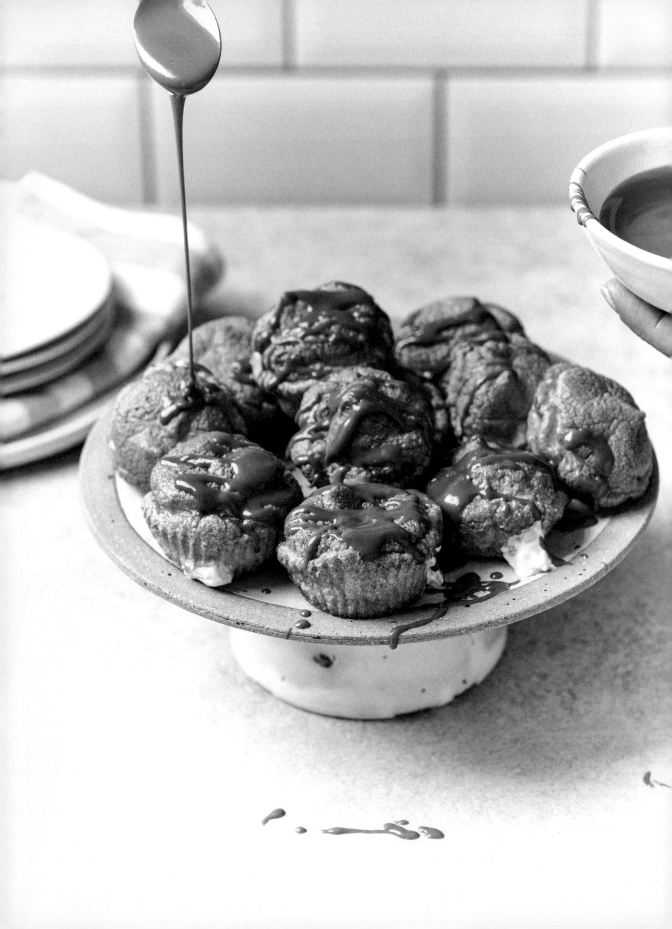

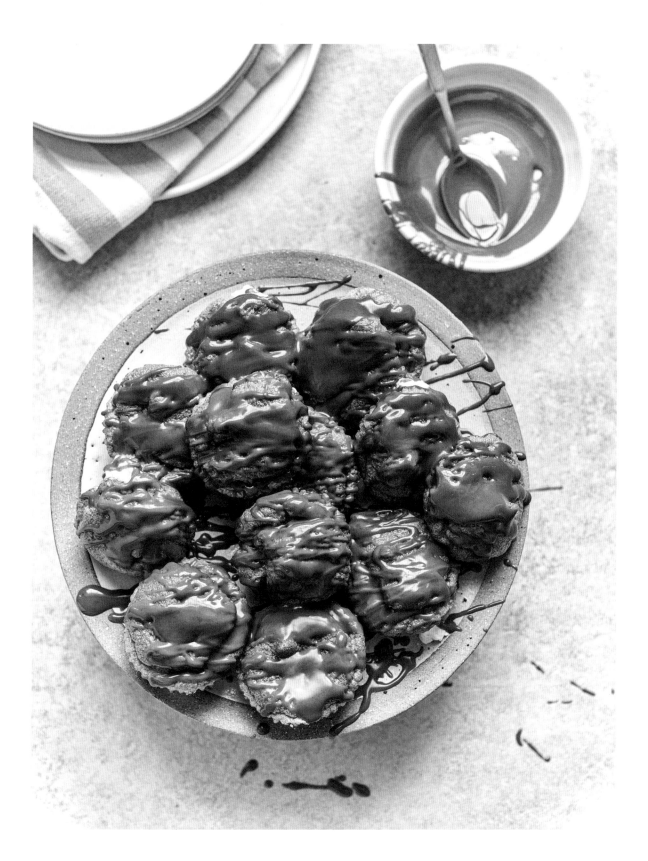

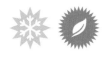

GOLDEN SYRUP LOAF CAKE

SERVES 12
PREP TIME: 12 MINUTES
COOK TIME: 1 HOUR 5 MINUTES

50g (1¾oz) butter
200g (7oz) golden syrup
25g (1oz) caster sugar
25g (1oz) dark brown soft sugar
2 eggs
80g (2¾oz) fat-free Greek yogurt
150ml (¼ pint) semi-skimmed milk
1 teaspoon vanilla extract
200g (7oz) self-raising flour
½ teaspoon baking powder

This was one of my childhood favourites. The recipe here is more modest in calories than the version of my childhood, but it still makes a delicious, moist loaf cake.

1   Preheat the oven to 160°C/140°C fan (325°F), Gas Mark 3. Line a 900g (2lb) loaf tin with nonstick baking paper, or a loaf tin liner.

2   In a small saucepan, melt together the butter, golden syrup and both types of sugar until everything is liquid, then set aside to cool slightly.

3   In a bowl, whisk the eggs with the yogurt, milk and vanilla extract.

4   Put the flour and baking powder in a mixing bowl, then pour over the syrup mixture and mix into the flour. Pour in the egg mixture, then stir to fully combine all the ingredients.

5   Carefully pour the batter into the prepared tin, using a spatula to scrape it out. Place on the middle shelf of the oven and bake for 1 hour.

6   Remove from the oven and allow to cool for 10 minutes before slicing.

PER SLICE
CALORIES 181
FAT 4.7G
SAT FAT 2.6G
CARBS 30G
SUGARS 18G
FIBRE 0.7G
PROTEIN 4G
SALT 0.44G

Note

If you want to add a little glaze to the cake, then, when it comes out of the oven, finely prick it all over with a fork. Heat up 2 tablespoons golden syrup in a pan and drizzle all over the top of the cake. Allow to cool for 10 minutes before serving.

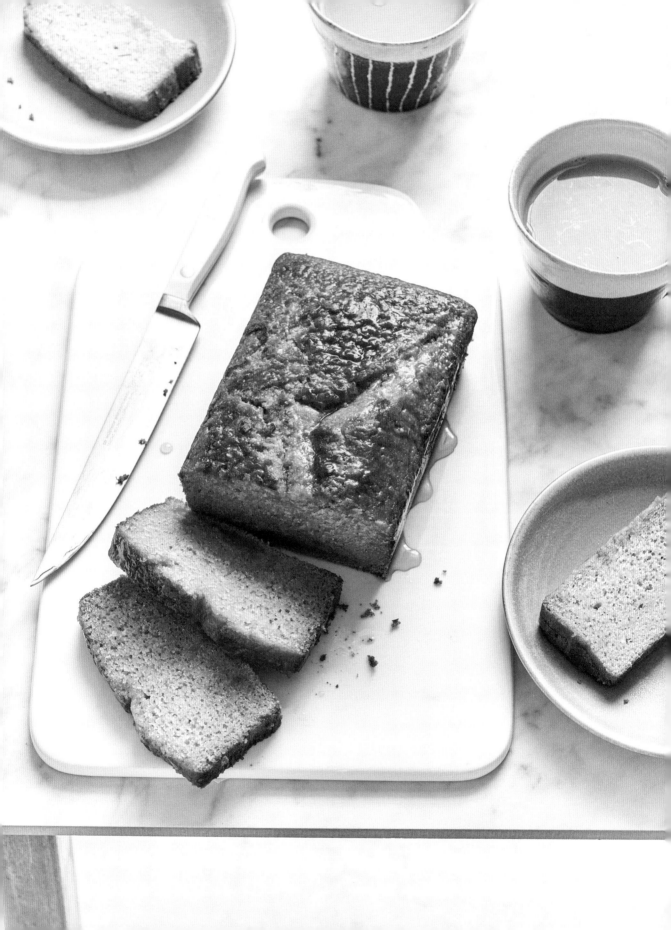

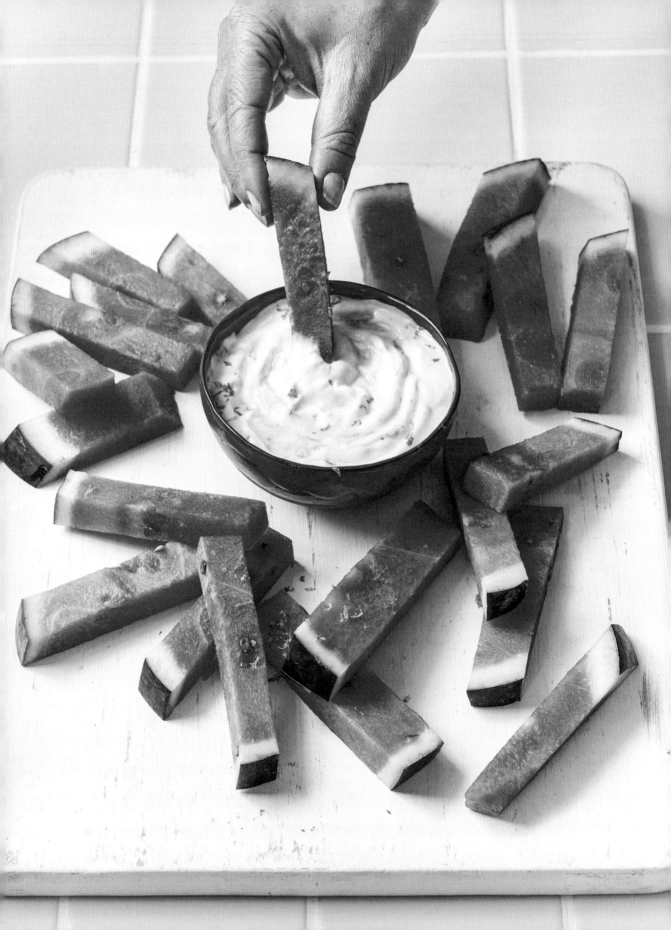

WATERMELON FINGERS WITH HONEY LIME DIP

SERVES 8
PREP TIME: 10 MINUTES
COOK TIME: NONE

1 watermelon
150g (5½oz) fat-free Greek yogurt
2 tablespoons honey
finely grated zest and juice of 1 lime

This is one of the most refreshing things I've eaten, so it's perfect for a hot summer's day, or a light post-barbecue dessert. Crisp, cold and refreshing watermelon dipped in a tangy and sweet lime dip really is a match made in heaven!

1   Slice the watermelon into fingers (see note below), keeping the rind on to make them easier to hold.

2   In a small bowl, mix the yogurt, honey, lime zest and juice.

3   Arrange the watermelon fingers on a platter and serve alongside the dip.

PER SERVING
CALORIES 138
FAT 1.1G
SAT FAT 0G
CARBS 26G
SUGARS 26G
FIBRE 1.7G
PROTEIN 3.4G
SALT TRACE

Note

To cut a watermelon into fingers, rinse it under cold running water and wipe off any dirt. On a chopping board, use a large, sharp knife to carefully cut the watermelon in half. Turn one half of the watermelon flat side down on the chopping board. Slice vertically down through the watermelon, from one side to the other, cutting slices about 2cm (¾ inch) wide. Turn the melon halfway, keeping the slices together, then cut across in the opposite direction, making square shapes on the rind. Voilà: watermelon fingers!

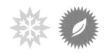

GINGERBREAD TREACLE MUFFINS

MAKES 4
PREP TIME: 10 MINUTES
COOK TIME: 18 MINUTES

low-calorie cooking spray
   (optional)
40g (1½oz) black treacle
40g (1½oz) honey
2 large eggs
30g (1oz) fat-free Greek yogurt
25ml (1fl oz) semi-skimmed milk
4 Weetabix, or other wheat biscuit
   cereal (total weight 80g / 2¾oz)
50g (1¾oz) self-raising flour
1 teaspoon baking powder
2 teaspoons ground ginger
½ teaspoon mixed spice
pinch of salt
60g (2¼oz) raisins

Warming gingerbread and mixed spice-scented muffins, made with wheat biscuit cereal for extra fibre. These are best eaten warm, fresh from the oven, but can still be enjoyed cold, or warmed up in the microwave and served with hot custard.

1   Preheat the oven to 200°C/180°C fan (400°F), Gas Mark 6. Place 4 nonstick paper muffin cases in a muffin tin. If your muffin cases are not nonstick, spray the insides all over with low-calorie cooking spray.

2   Put the treacle and honey in a small saucepan and heat through until the mixture begins to boil. Turn off the heat and allow to cool a little while you prepare the rest of the ingredients, but don't allow it to solidify.

3   Whisk together the eggs, yogurt and milk in a mixing bowl, then, with your hands, crush the cereal into fine crumbs into the bowl, then add the flour, baking powder, ginger, mixed spice and salt.

4   Pour the treacle mixture into the egg mixture and quickly stir it through the other ingredients. Add the raisins and mix again.

5   Divide the mixture between the muffin cases. If any raisins are sticking out of the batter, use a finger to poke them in a bit deeper. Place on the middle shelf of the oven and bake for 15 minutes.

6   After 15 minutes the muffins should be cooked through, fluffy in the middle and nicely browned (not burned) on top.

PER MUFFIN
CALORIES 268
FAT 3.5G
SAT FAT 1G
CARBS 48G
SUGARS 26G
FIBRE 3.4G
PROTEIN 8.9G
SALT 0.73G

Note

For a bit of crunch, add some chopped walnuts or pecans too.

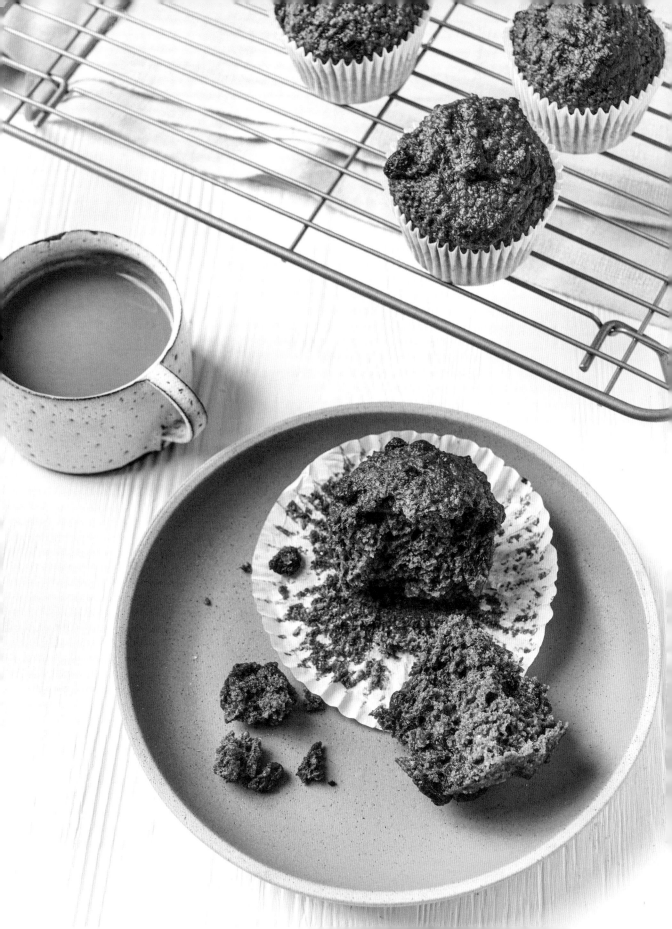

SCHOOL-STYLE CHOCOLATE CRACKNELL

MAKES 16 SQUARES
PREP TIME: 10 MINUTES
COOK TIME: NONE

175g (6oz) golden syrup

30g (1oz) butter

100g (3½oz) Rice Krispies, or other crispy puff rice cereal

75g (2¾oz) dried skimmed milk powder

25g (1oz) cocoa powder

Do you remember this from your school days? A classic school dessert which was actually really good! My youngest daughter came home talking about it, so we decided to make our own slightly lower-sugar version. This is a great treat to make with kids.

1   Line a 20cm (8 inch) square baking tin with nonstick baking paper.

2   Melt the golden syrup and butter together in a small saucepan and allow to bubble for 1 minute, being careful that it doesn't bubble up over the edge of the pan.

3   Tip the Rice Krispies or cereal into a mixing bowl and add the milk powder and cocoa powder. Mix them together thoroughly.

4   Pour in the syrup mixture and quickly and thoroughly mix everything together.

5   Scoop the mixture into the prepared tin. Use a wooden spoon to pat it down firmly and evenly into the tin.

6   Leave it to cool and set – this should only take about 30 minutes.

7   Remove from the tin and use a sharp knife to cut it into 16 pieces.

PER SQUARE
CALORIES 94
FAT 2G
SAT FAT 1.2G
CARBS 16G
SUGARS 11G
FIBRE 0.5G
PROTEIN 2.5G
SALT 0.23G

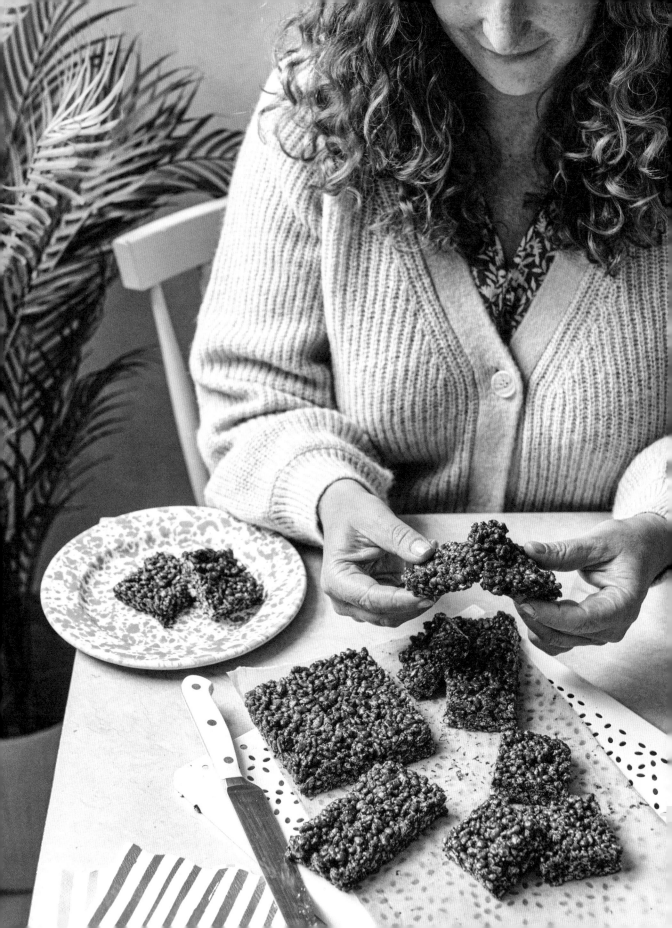

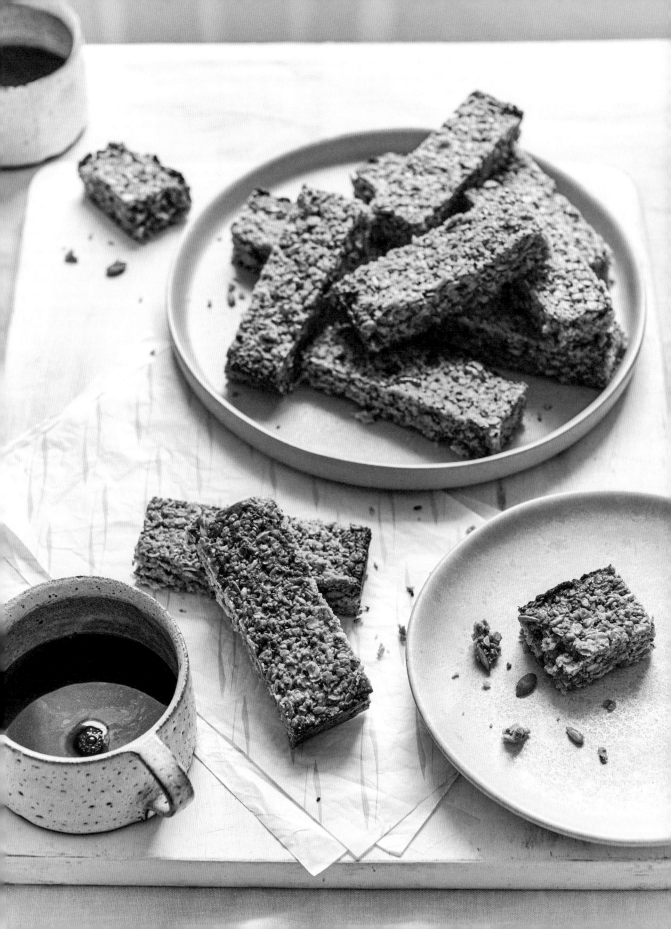

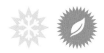

JUST-RIGHT FLAPJACKS

MAKES 12
PREP TIME: 10 MINUTES
COOK TIME: 20 MINUTES

100g (3½oz) butter
100g (3½oz) honey
45g (1½oz) dark brown soft sugar
300g (10½oz) fine porridge oats
25g (1oz) sunflower seeds
25g (1oz) pumpkin seeds
2 tablespoons chia seeds
2 eggs, lightly beaten
1 teaspoon vanilla extract
pinch of salt

I've tried so many flapjack recipes and it always feels like a bit of a Goldilocks experience: too hard, too soft, too crumbly... The other thing about flapjacks is that, although they appear to be a 'healthy' sweet treat, they generally have an awful lot of sugar and butter holding them together. These are my compromise: crunchy without being tooth breaking, sweet without overkill, while a mix of seeds alongside the oats gives them a bit of extra crunch as well as additional vitamins and minerals.

These are delicious either warm or cold and will last up to 5 days in an airtight container: perfect for snacks and packed lunches.

1   Preheat the oven to 200°C/180°C fan (350°F), Gas Mark 4. Line a 20cm (8 inch) square baking tin with nonstick baking paper.

2   In a medium-sized pan, melt the butter, honey and sugar together. Stir together to form a syrup.

3   Remove the pan from the heat and add the oats and seeds, stirring and mixing well to fully coat the oats. Leave to cool a little.

4   Stir the beaten eggs thoroughly into the flapjack mixture.

5   Scrape the mixture into the prepared tin, then press it firmly and evenly into the tin. I use a square of baking paper to do this by hand, so I can feel if any parts are much thicker than others and even out the surface.

6   Bake on the middle shelf of the oven for 18 minutes. Allow to cool for 15 minutes before removing from the tin and cutting into 12 slices. To do this, cut into 4 even pieces one way, then 3 even pieces the other way.

PER FLAPJACK
CALORIES 246
FAT 12G
SAT FAT 5.2G
CARBS 27G
SUGARS 10G
FIBRE 2.9G
PROTEIN 5.6G
SALT 0.23G

Note

I keep these nut-free so my daughters can take them into school in their packed lunches, but broken-up nuts such as walnuts, pecans, hazelnuts and peanuts all add extra crunch and flavour. You can also add 1 teaspoon ground cinnamon or mixed spice. I sometimes add chocolate chips, or cover the flapjacks with a drizzle of melted chocolate for the kids.

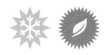

BLUEBERRY SCONES

MAKES 12
PREP TIME: 15 MINUTES
COOK TIME: 15 MINUTES

500g (1lb 2oz) plain flour, plus more if needed and to dust

1 tablespoon baking powder

2 tablespoons caster sugar

¼ teaspoon fine salt

50g (1¾oz) butter, cut into small pieces

60g (2¼oz) fat-free Greek yogurt

2 eggs

about 250ml (9fl oz) milk, or a little more, as needed

1 teaspoon vanilla extract

150g (5½oz) fresh blueberries

I had no idea that these were a classic Lake District bakery treat until I visited with friends a few years ago, where we ate the most gorgeous blueberry scones. They make a lovely home-baked treat too. I serve them with butter or jam (or both) and they always go down a treat with my family.

1 Preheat the oven to 220°C/200°C fan (425°F), Gas Mark 7. Line a baking tray with nonstick baking paper.

2 Pour the flour, baking powder, caster sugar and salt into a mixing bowl, add the butter and yogurt, then use your fingers to rub them into the flour, breaking up the clumps of butter and turning the mixture into something resembling crumbs.

3 Lightly beat one of the eggs in a measuring jug, then pour in enough milk to make the level up to 300ml (½ pint). Add the vanilla extract and mix.

4 Stir the blueberries into the dry mixture. Pour the milk and egg mixture into the bowl and use a table knife to mix everything together. I stir it around the bowl in a stirring and scooping motion, to bring the wet and dry elements together. If you use your hands at this point, more will end up on your hands than anywhere else. If it's too sticky, add a little more flour.

5 Once you have a rough dough, you can go in with your hands to fully bring it all together into a smoother dough. Now divide the dough in half, roll the first half into a ball, place on a floured work surface and use your hand to press down on it to form a disc about 3cm (1¼ inches) thick.

6 Now use a sharp knife to cut the disc in half to form a semicircle, then cut each semi-circle into 3 to form pie-like slices. Repeat this with the other ball of dough. You should end up with 12 scones.

7 Transfer the scones to the prepared tray, leaving space between each one. Beat the other egg in a small bowl and use a pastry brush to brush a little egg over the top of each scone.

8 Place on the middle shelf of the oven and bake for 15 minutes. By this time, they should have risen impressively and turned a rich golden brown on top. These will keep in an airtight container for up to 3 days, or you can freeze them too.

PER SCONE
CALORIES 221
FAT 5.2G
SAT FAT 2.8G
CARBS 36G
SUGARS 4.7G
FIBRE 1.9G
PROTEIN 6.8G
SALT 0.54G

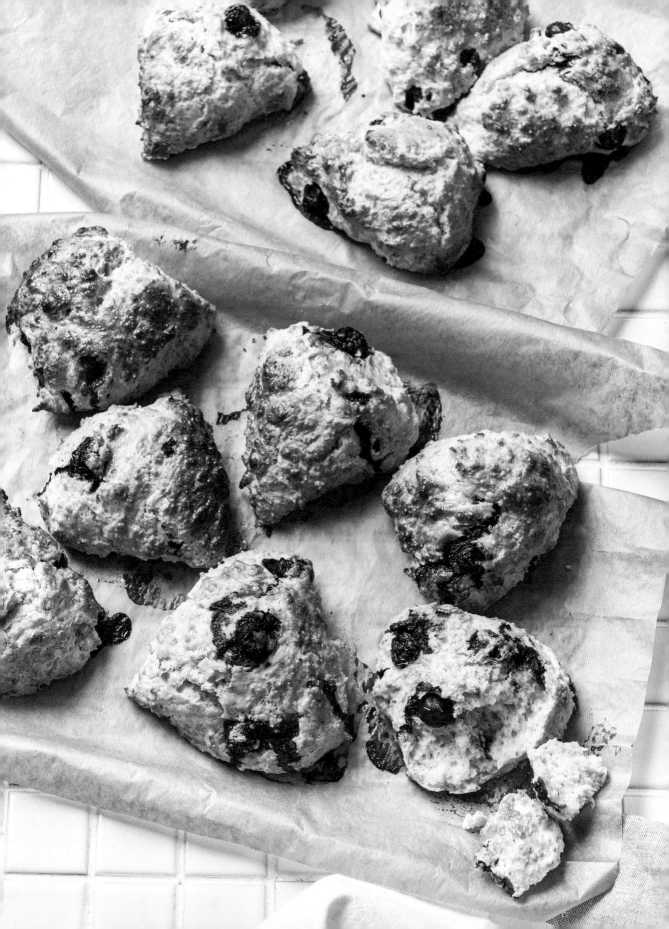

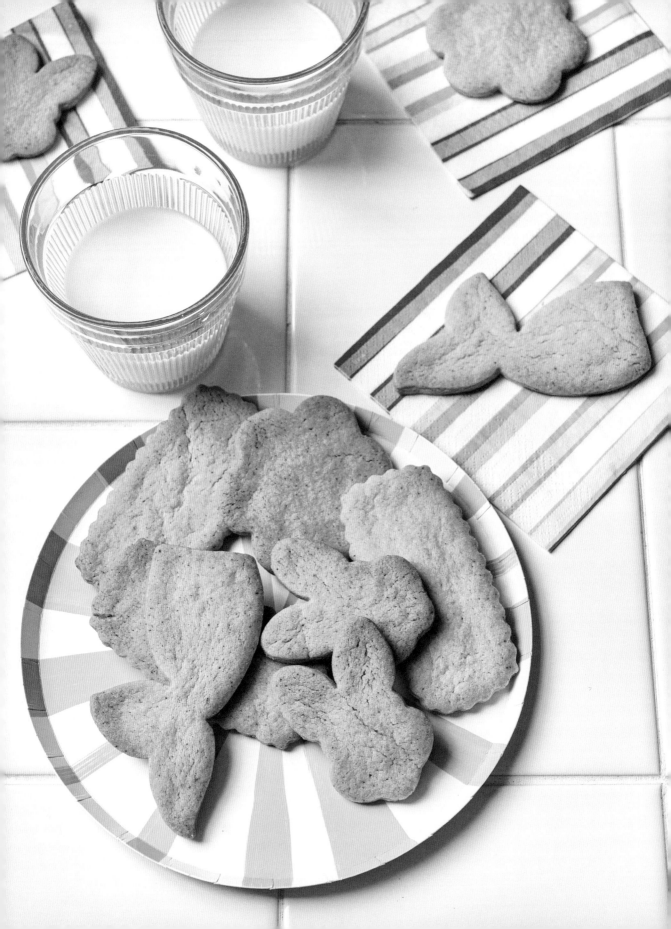

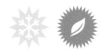

SHREWSBURY BISCUITS

MAKES 28 (DEPENDING ON WHAT SHAPE CUTTER YOU USE)
PREP TIME: 15 MINUTES
COOK TIME: 12–15 MINUTES

110g (4oz) baking spread

110g (4oz) caster sugar

1 egg yolk

pinch of fine salt

225g (8oz) self-raising flour, plus more to dust

finely grated zest of 1 lemon

I used to spend a lot of time at my friend Charlotte's house when I was at primary school and I still have a little handwritten recipe from Charlotte's mum, Janet, with 'Pippa's favourite' written next to it. I can clearly remember Janet baking these, with the most delicious smell filling the house. She would also bake them in cute shapes, which made them all the more appealing. I hadn't made the recipe for many years, but I recently baked them for my own girls and they were just as good as I remember. A great, simple cookie recipe to have on hand. Even better if they are baked into the shapes of cute animals!

1   Preheat the oven to 180°C/160°C fan (350°F), Gas Mark 4. Line a large baking tray, or 2 smaller trays, with nonstick baking paper.

2   In a mixing bowl, cream the baking spread and sugar together and beat until pale and soft. Add the egg yolk, salt and 1 tablespoon of the flour and beat again.

3   Add the remaining flour and the lemon zest and stir to bring together into a dough.

4   On a floured work surface, roll the biscuit dough out thinly, to about 5mm (¼ inch) thick. Cut into shapes, lay on the prepared tray or trays, then bake for 12–15 minutes, until a light golden brown.

5   Allow to cool on the trays for a few minutes, before transferring to a cooling rack.

PER BISCUIT
CALORIES 71
FAT 3.1G
SAT FAT 0.7G
CARBS 9.8G
SUGARS 4G
FIBRE 0.5G
PROTEIN 0.9G
SALT 0.13G

Note

These are great to make with kids, as there is no need to chill the dough before cooking – so little patience is required – and because they don't spread they hold their shape when baking, which means you can use novelty cutters! They will keep for up to 1 week in an airtight container.

- ✓ COUSCOUS WITH A CRUNCH
- ✓ GREEN BEANS WITH SPRING ONIONS AND GARLIC
- ✓ ZAKKOKU RICE
- ✓ ROASTED RADISHES
- ✓ SESAME SHREDDED CARROT SALAD
- ✓ SALT AND VINEGAR ROAST POTATOES
- ✓ BOULANGÈRE POTATOES
- ✓ SPINACH, LIME AND JALAPEÑO DIP
- ✓ FRIED CHEESE `CROUTONS`
- ✓ SCOTTISH OATCAKES
- ✓ EVERYTHING SEASONING
- ✓ INDIAN 5-SPICE BLEND
- ✓ RAS EL HANOUT SPICE MIX

9

Lucky Dip

COUSCOUS WITH A CRUNCH

SERVES 6
PREP TIME: 5 MINUTES
COOK TIME: 5 MINUTES

300g (10½oz) wholewheat
    couscous
500ml (18fl oz) boiling-hot chicken
    stock
50g (1¾oz) flaked almonds
finely grated zest of 1 lemon, plus
    1 tablespoon lemon juice
2 large handfuls of mint leaves,
    finely chopped

Just a couple of simple additions to couscous can transform it from a slightly boring side dish into a tasty addition to any meal. The great thing about couscous is that it's so quick to make, so if you've put all your effort into the accompanying dish, you can quickly whip this up just before serving. Using hot stock instead of freshly boiled water is a great way to instantly add more flavour. Here I've used chopped mint leaves and toasted flaked almonds to bring it up a level, but other chopped herbs – added once the couscous is ready – work brilliantly, too. Try serving this with Chicken Tagine (see page 147).

1   Place the couscous in a saucepan or bowl, pour over the boiling-hot stock and cover with a lid or a plate. Set a timer for 5 minutes while you prepare the other ingredients.

2   Toast the flaked almonds in a small dry frying pan until they start to turn a golden-brown colour and you can smell the toasty fragrance. Just shuffle them around with a wooden spoon, or shake the pan, every 15 seconds or so. It should only take 3–4 minutes over a medium heat. Keep an eye on them to make sure they don't catch and burn and remove from the heat as soon as they are done.

3   After the couscous has soaked in the stock for 5 minutes, add the lemon zest, lemon juice and mint and mix everything up using a fork.

4   Scatter the toasted almonds over the couscous to serve.

PER SERVING
CALORIES 241
FAT 5.9G
SAT FAT 0.7G
CARBS 34G
SUGARS 2.3G
FIBRE 5.7G
PROTEIN 10G
SALT 0.48G

Note

To make this vegetarian, simply use vegetable stock rather than chicken stock.

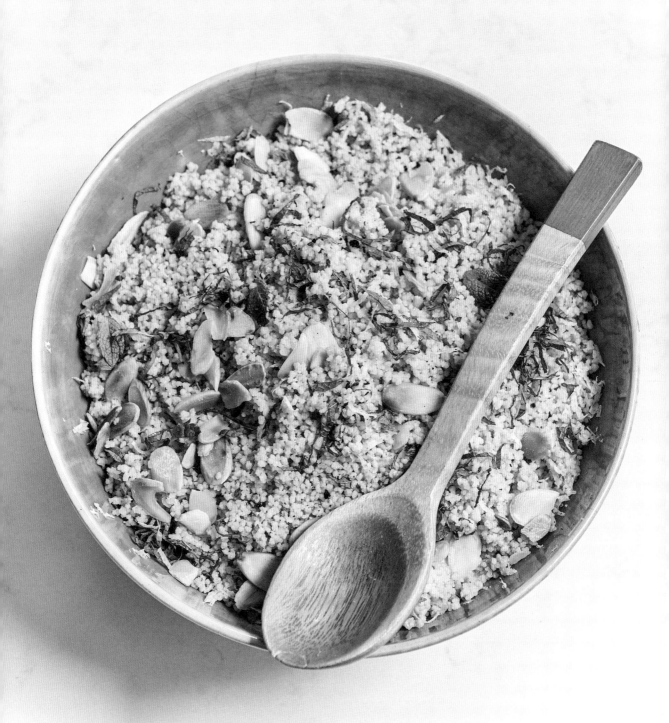

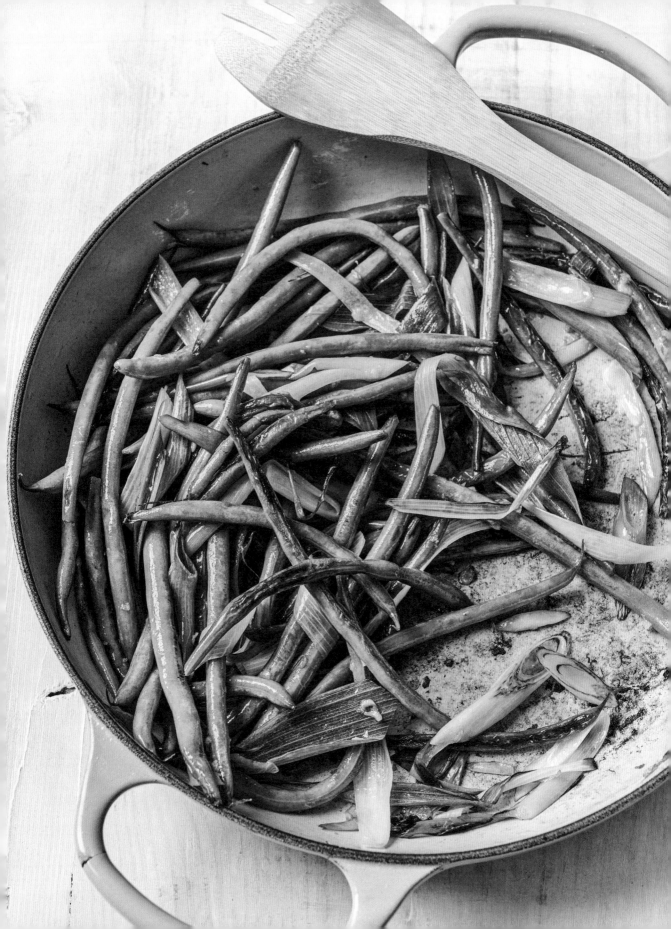

GREEN BEANS WITH SPRING ONIONS & GARLIC

SERVES 4
PREP TIME: 5 MINUTES
COOK TIME: 10 MINUTES

1 teaspoon olive oil

300g (10½oz) green beans, trimmed and cut into 3–4cm (1¼–1½ inch) pieces

8 spring onions, sliced

1 large garlic clove, crushed

salt and pepper

Level up green beans with this simple combination. They make a brilliant accompaniment to most main meals; I like to serve them with my Beef & Stout Hotpot (see page 183).

1   Heat the oil in a frying pan over a medium-high heat, add the green beans and spring onions and stir-fry for 9 minutes. A little bit of charring on the beans is encouraged here, but avoid burning them.

2   Reduce the heat to low, add the garlic to the pan and stir-fry for 1 more minute. Remove from the heat, season with salt and pepper and serve.

PER SERVING
CALORIES 39
FAT 1.5G
SAT FAT 0.2G
CARBS 3G
SUGARS 2.2G
FIBRE 3.1G
PROTEIN 2G
SALT 0.25G

ZAKKOKU RICE

MAKES 12 PORTIONS
PREP TIME: 2 MINUTES
COOK TIME: 10 MINUTES

400g (14oz) sushi rice

200g (7oz) quinoa (any type will do, but I prefer mixed colours for this)

150g (5½oz) bulgur wheat

150g (5½oz) buckwheat

4 tablespoons poppy seeds

This is a Japanese style of rice, which is bolstered with other grains and seeds. One of its beauties is that it's a great way of using up bits and pieces leftover in packets, while making a simple rice side dish into something so much more interesting. You really can customize it to your own tastes, or to what happens to need using up in your store cupboard. I make up the grain and seed mixture, store it in a large, airtight container and then have it handy for using when I want a side dish that's a little more interesting than plain rice.

1   Simply mix all the ingredients and transfer into an airtight storage container.

2   When I am ready to use this, I allow 75g (2¾oz) per person and double the amount of water. So, for 75g (2¾oz) of rice mix, use 150ml (¼ pint) of water; for 150g (5½oz) rice, use 300ml (½ pint) water and so on.

3   Place in a small saucepan which has a lid, cover with the water and bring to a simmer. Cover with a lid and simmer for 10 minutes, then turn off the heat and leave to rest for 10 minutes, still with the lid on. Fluff through with a fork and serve.

PER SERVING
CALORIES 280
FAT 3G
SAT FAT 0.4G
CARBS 54G
SUGARS 0.5G
FIBRE 3G
PROTEIN 7.9G
SALT TRACE

Note

Other ideas for what to add to a zakkoku mix: long grain and basmati rice, oats, linseeds, sesame seeds, flaxseeds, aramanth... experiment to find your favourite combination!

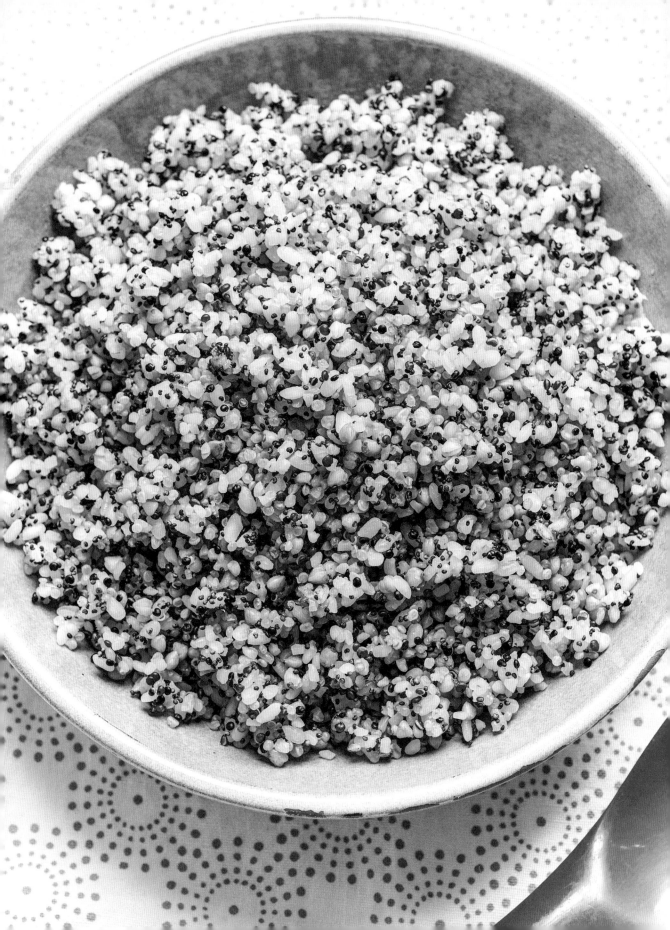

ROASTED RADISHES

SERVES 4
PREP TIME: 10 MINUTES
COOK TIME: 25 MINUTES

Radishes are great value when they are in season in the UK, and roasting them gives them a tender consistency which makes a lovely, unusual side dish with a roast dinner.

400g (14oz) radishes, ends trimmed
½ tablespoon melted butter
½ teaspoon coarse ground salt
¼ teaspoon dried parsley
¼ teaspoon dried dill
a few grinds of black pepper
2 garlic cloves, crushed

1   Preheat the oven to 220°C/200°C fan (425°F), Gas Mark 7.

2   Tip the radishes into a small baking tray or ovenproof dish with the butter, salt, parsley, dill and pepper and mix together thoroughly.

3   Bake for 20 minutes, giving them a toss halfway through cooking.

4   Take them out of the oven, stir through the crushed garlic, then bake for another 5 minutes. They should be light golden brown, with a tender consistency. Serve.

PER SERVING
CALORIES 30
FAT 1.8G
SAT FAT 1.1G
CARBS 2.3G
SUGARS 1.9G
FIBRE 1G
PROTEIN 0.7G
SALT 0.68G

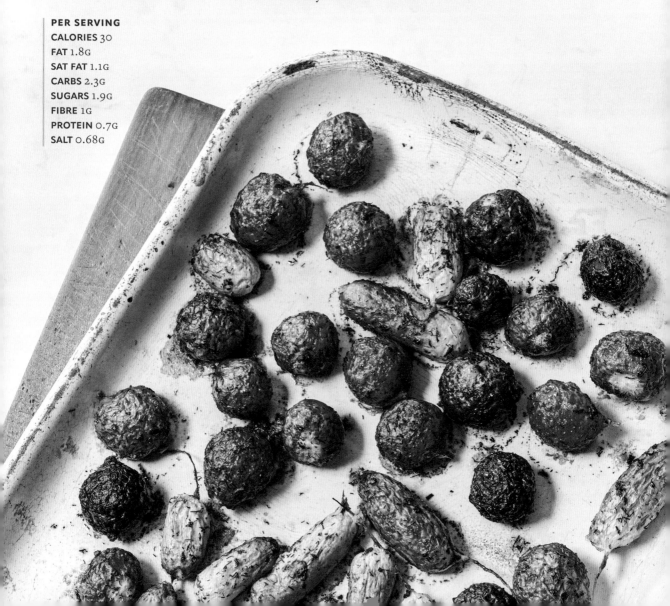

SESAME SHREDDED CARROT SALAD

SERVES 4
PREP TIME: 10 MINUTES
COOK TIME: NONE

500g (1lb 2oz) carrots, coarsely grated or julienned (see recipe introduction)
1 tablespoon rice vinegar
1 teaspoon sesame oil
1 teaspoon light soy sauce
1 tablespoon sesame seeds

PER SERVING
CALORIES 84
FAT 3.1G
SAT FAT 0.6G
CARBS 9.9G
SUGARS 9.2G
FIBRE 5.1G
PROTEIN 1.2G
SALT 0.29G

This is an easy and cheap salad to knock up and it works perfectly alongside gyoza (for homemade, see page 150), noodles and rice dishes. The quickest way to grate the carrots is using a mandoline, or the grater attachment on a food processor, but you can also get great results using a julienne peeler or the larger holes on a box grater.

1 Place all the ingredients into a large bowl and toss well to coat the carrots. Serve.

Note

Try adding grated beetroot, radishes, or – for a bit of green – some thinly sliced spring onions or finely chopped parsley leaves.

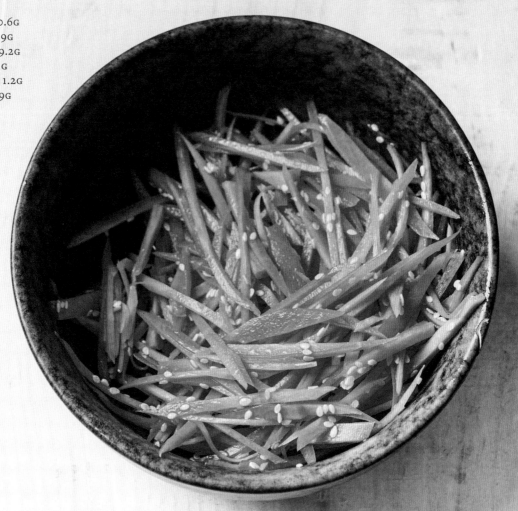

SALT & VINEGAR ROAST POTATOES

SERVES 4
PREP TIME: 10 MINUTES
COOK TIME: 1 HOUR 5 MINUTES

1kg (2lb 4oz) potatoes, such as Maris Piper, cut into chunks (medium potatoes into 4, large potatoes into 6)
300ml (½ pint) distilled white vinegar
500ml (18fl oz) cold water
2 tablespoons olive oil
1 tablespoon sea salt flakes
freshly ground black pepper

If you love salt and vinegar crisps, you are sure to love these salt and vinegar roast potatoes. They are a great twist to have alongside a classic roast dinner.

1   Put the potato chunks in a large saucepan and cover them with the vinegar and measured cold water. Bring to the boil, cover with a lid, then simmer for 20 minutes.

2   Preheat the oven to 220°C/200°C fan (425°F), Gas Mark 7.

3   Drain the potatoes and leave them in the colander to steam dry for 10 minutes.

4   In the saucepan, or a bowl, gently stir the potatoes together with the oil, salt and pepper (being careful not to break them apart).

5   Tip into a roasting tin and roast for 40–45 minutes until crisp and golden brown.

PER SERVING
CALORIES 255
FAT 6.5G
SAT FAT 0.9G
CARBS 42G
SUGARS 1.8G
FIBRE 3G
PROTEIN 5G
SALT 1.7G

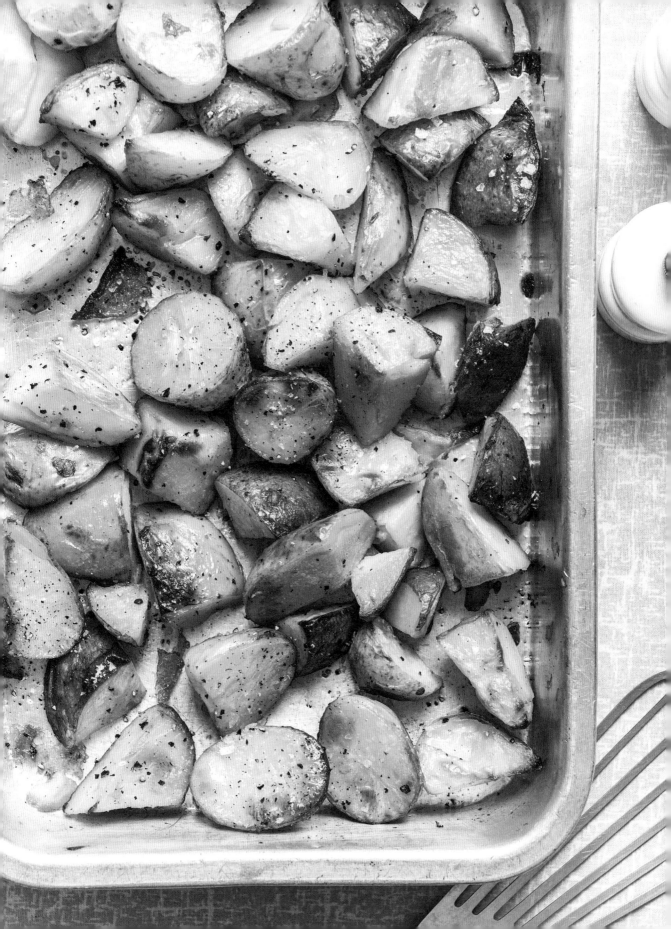

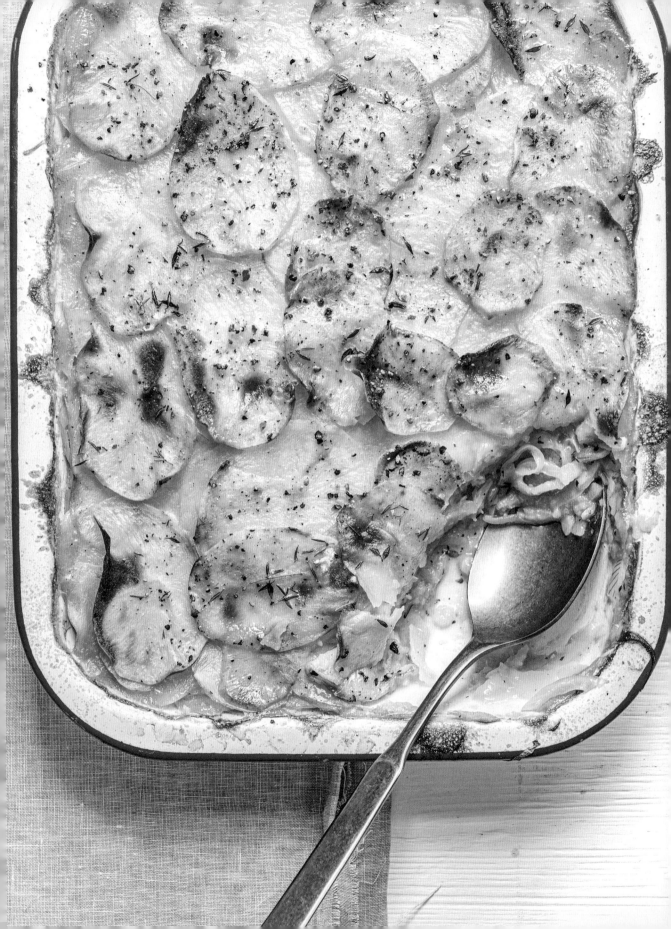

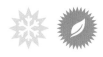

BOULANGÈRE POTATOES

SERVES 6
PREP TIME: 15 MINUTES
COOK TIME: 1 HOUR

1.5kg (3lb 5oz) Maris Piper potatoes
1 tablespoon butter
2 onions, finely sliced
2 garlic cloves, crushed
3 thyme sprigs, leaves removed
400ml (14fl oz) hot vegetable stock
spray oil, or low calorie cooking spray
salt and pepper

These are a great alternative to roast potatoes. Once the initial preparation is done, they are very low maintenance, as you just leave them cooking in the oven, which is perfect if you have something else in there already. They make a great accompaniment to the Pot-Roast Beef with Red Wine Gravy, Beef & Stout Hotpot, or Slow-Cooker Mushroom Bourguignon (see pages 179, 183 and 175).

1   Preheat the oven to 200°C/180°C fan (400°F), Gas Mark 6.

2   Peel and slice the potatoes as thinly as you can (you can use a mandoline or a food processor attachment for this).

3   Melt the butter in a frying pan over a medium-low heat and fry the onions for 10 minutes until they are soft and golden, adding the garlic for the last minute of cooking.

4   Arrange one-third of the potatoes in a single layer in an ovenproof dish (I use a rectangular dish measuring 30 x 20cm / 12 x 8 inches). Add half the fried onions and garlic, spreading them around evenly. Scatter over a few thyme leaves and season with a few grinds of salt and pepper.

5   Now add another layer of potatoes, the rest of the onions, more thyme, salt and pepper, then the final layer of potatoes. Pour the vegetable stock evenly over the top, then finally season with a little more salt and pepper and a few more thyme leaves. Spray the top with spray oil, or low-calorie cooking spray, then place on the middle shelf of the oven to bake for 50 minutes.

6   When you remove the dish from the oven, the potatoes should be tender, with a golden colour on top and some darker crispy edges. Allow to rest for 5 minutes before serving.

PER SERVING
CALORIES 245
FAT 2.9G
SAT FAT 1.4G
CARBS 47G
SUGARS 4.9G
FIBRE 4.1G
PROTEIN 5.6G
SALT 0.33G

Note

You can replace some of the regular potato with a layer of sweet potato, or thin slices of butternut squash, for some variety. You can also change the herbs you use in order to complement different meals: rosemary and sage also work well. A few fennel seeds fried in with the onions adds another level of depth to the flavour, while some finely grated Parmesan cheese sprinkled between layers and on top of the potatoes also makes a delicious addition.

SPINACH, LIME & JALAPEÑO DIP

SERVES 4
PREP TIME: 5 MINUTES
COOK TIME: NONE

This is a great quick and easy side or dip, which I use as an alternative to guacamole. It complements Mexican and Tex-Mex meals such as fajitas, burritos and chilli con carne.

2 large handfuls of baby spinach
    leaves

400g (14oz) can of cannellini
    beans, drained

3 tablespoons fat-free Greek yogurt

1 tablespoon pickled jalapeños

1 garlic clove

1 teaspoon coarse ground salt

finely grated zest and juice of 1 lime

1   Place all the ingredients into a mini chopper or blender and whizz together until smooth in consistency.

PER SERVING
CALORIES 93
FAT 0.5G
SAT FAT 0G
CARBS 11G
SUGARS 1.5G
FIBRE 5G
PROTEIN 8G
SALT 1.5G

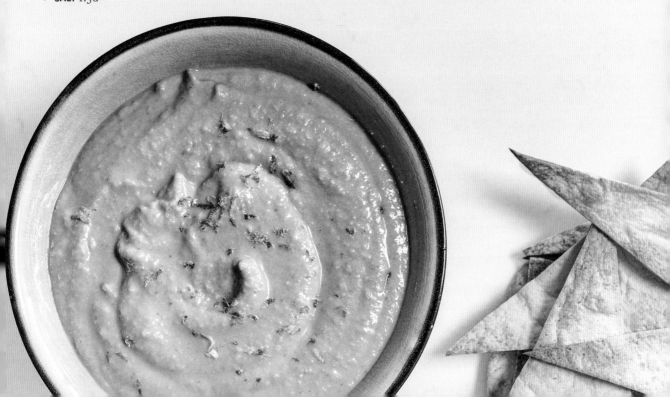

FRIED CHEESE 'CROUTONS'

SERVES 4
PREP TIME: 2 MINUTES
COOK TIME: 15 MINUTES

120g (4½oz) Cheddar cheese, grated

PER SERVING
CALORIES 124
FAT 10G
SAT FAT 6.5G
CARBS 0G
SUGARS 0G
FIBRE 0G
PROTEIN 7.5G
SALT 0.54G

You know those little bits of crispy golden cheese on the edge of the cheese toastie which are always the tastiest bit? How about creating a giant, crisp, golden bit of cheese that you can snap apart to make crunchy, delicious croutons? This is a great way to top off soups, salads, pasta dishes... just a little sprinkling of these adds a crunchy burst of flavour.

1 Spread the grated cheese evenly over the bottom of a nonstick frying pan, set over a medium heat and watch the cheese melt.

2 Increase the heat a little and let the cheese bubble away until it forms into a golden-hued crust that you can lift at the edges. There's a fine line between lightly toasting this and letting it burn, so keep an eye on it, move the pan around if you get hotspots on your hob, then remove the pan from the heat once you have a golden-brown colour and a slightly harder consistency. This will take 10–15 minutes.

3 Remove the pan from the heat source and allow the cheese to cool before lifting it out and laying it on a piece of kitchen paper to absorb the excess fat. Once cooled, you should be able to snap it apart into smaller pieces. Store in an airtight container for up to 3 days.

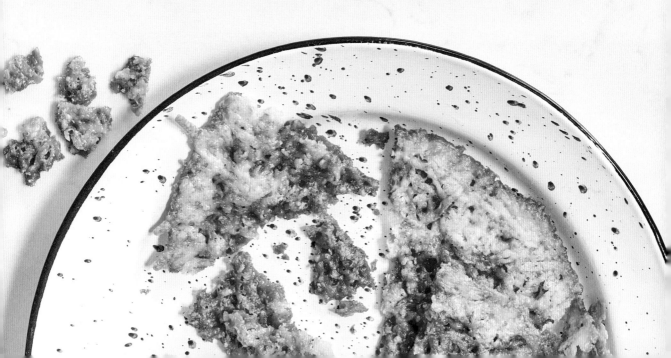

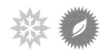

SCOTTISH OATCAKES

MAKES ABOUT 16
PREP TIME: 15 MINUTES
COOK TIME: 20 MINUTES

225g (8oz) fine oatmeal, plus more
to dust

¼ teaspoon bicarbonate of soda

¼ teaspoon fine salt

1 tablespoon (15g / ½oz) melted
butter

about 150ml (¼ pint) boiling water

These simple oat crackers make a great snack to serve with cheese, top with cream cheese and smoked salmon, or as a side to soup or Slow-Cooked Scottish Stovies with Brisket (see page 176).

1 Preheat the oven to 180°C/160°C fan (350°F), Gas Mark 4.

2 Put the oatmeal in a mixing bowl, add the bicarbonate of soda and salt, then mix in the melted butter.

3 Add about half the measured boiling water and use a palette knife or butter knife to incorporate it into the oat mixture, bringing it together to form a dough. Add more of the measured water a little at a time until you have a thick dough, but don't add too much or you will make it too sticky. Use your hands to roll the dough into a ball.

4 Scatter some oatmeal over a clean work surface, then use a rolling pin to roll the dough out to a thickness of about 5mm (¼ inch). Use a 6cm (2½ inch) fluted cutter to cut out the oatcakes, gathering up the offcuts and rolling it out again when you need to. This should make about 16 oatcakes.

5 Use a palette knife to gently lift the oatcakes on to a nonstick baking tray.

6 Bake them on the middle shelf of the oven for 20 minutes, turning them over halfway through, to allow them to crisp up on both sides.

PER OATCAKE
CALORIES 62
FAT 1.9G
SAT FAT 0.7G
CARBS 9G
SUGARS 0G
FIBRE 1.1G
PROTEIN 1.6G
SALT 0.13G

Note

You can store these in an airtight container for up to 5 days. You can also freeze them by layering them with nonstick baking paper and storing in a freezer bag or airtight container. The best way to defrost them is under a hot grill.

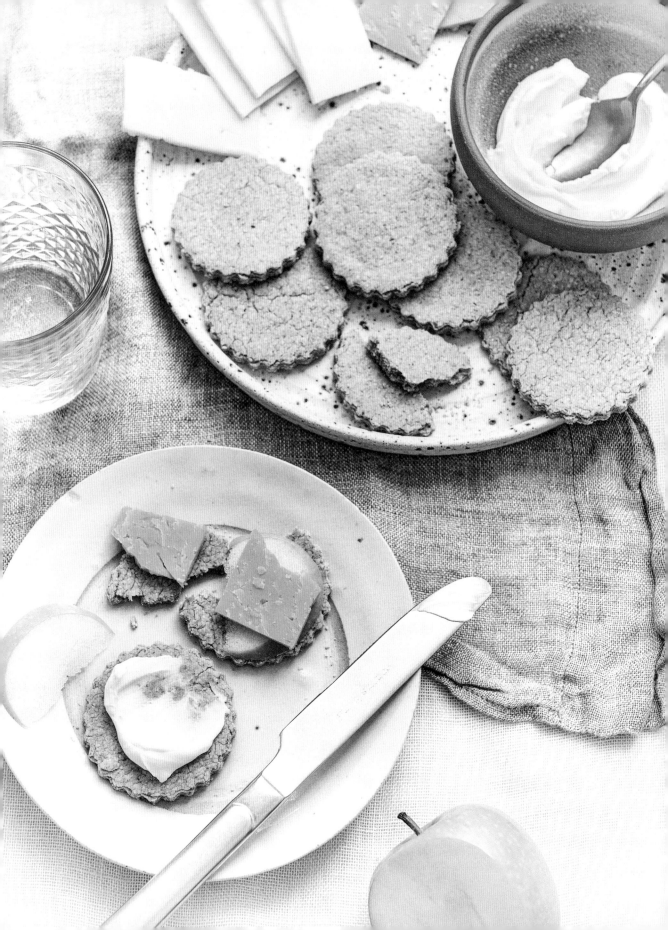

EVERYTHING SEASONING

MAKES 8 TABLESPOONS
PREP TIME: 5 MINUTES
COOK TIME: NONE

2 tablespoons poppy seeds
2½ tablespoon white sesame seeds
2 tablespoons black sesame seeds
   (or see recipe introduction)
½ tablespoon garlic granules
½ tablespoon onion granules
½ tablespoon fine salt

If you haven't tried an 'everything bagel', then you are missing out. Although there is some conflict over who invented them, they seem to have their roots in New York and the mixture is a really delicious combination. Although this seasoning mix is wonderful on a bagel, it can be used for so much more, so here is how to whip up your own batch! If you can't get hold of black sesame seeds, add an extra 1 tablespoon each of white sesame seeds and poppy seeds.

1   Pop everything in a jar and shake it up!

PER TABLESPOON
CALORIES 54
FAT 4.6G
SAT FAT 0.8G
CARBS 0.8G
SUGARS 0G
FIBRE 1G
PROTEIN 1.8G
SALT 0.3G

Note

Here are some ideas of what you can do with this seasoning:
> Add a crunchy coating to fish and meat.
> Stir into cream cheese to spread over plain bagels and serve with smoked salmon.
> Add to dips.
> Sprinkle over salads and coleslaws.
> Sprinkle over mac 'n' cheese.
> Use for my Everything Seasoned Dough Balls (see page 159).

INDIAN 5-SPICE BLEND

**MAKES ENOUGH FOR
6-8 MEALS**
PREP TIME: 2 MINUTES
COOK TIME: NONE

4 tablespoons cumin seeds
3 tablespoons brown mustard seeds
2 tablespoons fenugreek seeds
2 tablespoons nigella seeds
2 tablespoons fennel seeds

PER ⅛ OF A BATCH
CALORIES 47
FAT 2.5G
SAT FAT 0.2G
CARBS 2.3G
SUGARS 0G
FIBRE 1.9G
PROTEIN 2.9G
SALT TRACE

Known as *panch phoran*, this is a quick little blend of spices that you can throw together and can be used in a variety of ways for easy mealtimes. You can add it to basmati rice as it cooks, use it as a rub for meats, sprinkle it over curries as a garnish, or use it as a base spice mix for a curry, such as my Black Bean, Kale & Sweet Potato Curry (see page 24).

1   Simply measure the seeds into a dry frying pan, turn on the heat to medium and dry-fry them for a minute or so until they are lightly toasted (be aware that the mustard seeds may spit). Be careful not to burn them, but as they toast you should be able to smell their fragrance.

2   Allow them to cool, then transfer to a glass jar or airtight container.

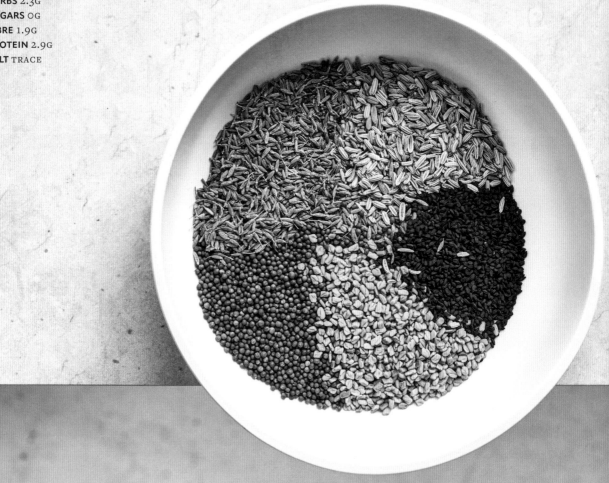

RAS EL HANOUT SPICE MIX

**MAKES ENOUGH FOR
4 MEALS**
PREP TIME: 5 MINUTES
COOK TIME: NONE

1 tablespoon ground cumin

1 tablespoon ground ginger

1 tablespoon sweet paprika

2 teaspoons fine salt

2 teaspoons freshly ground black
   pepper

2 teaspoons ground allspice

1 teaspoon ground cinnamon

1 teaspoon ground coriander

½ teaspoon ground cloves

½ teaspoon cayenne pepper

**A Middle-Eastern spice blend which can have many variations.
Here is my favourite homemade combination.**

1   Pop everything in a jar and shake it up!

PER ¼ BATCH SERVING
CALORIES 27
FAT 0.9G
SAT FAT 0.1G
CARBS 2.9G
SUGARS 0.7G
FIBRE 2G
PROTEIN 0.9G
SALT 2.5G

Note

You can tweak the flavours in this to your own taste. If you want a version that isn't spicy, omit the cayenne pepper.

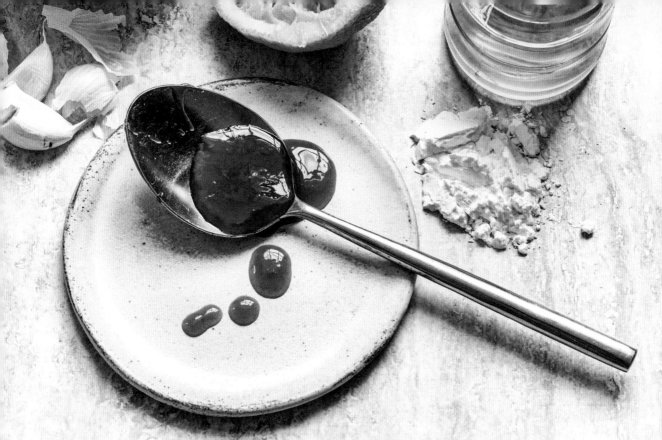

TERIYAKI SAUCE

MAKES 8 SERVINGS
PREP TIME: 5 MINUTES
COOK TIME: 12 MINUTES

80ml (3fl oz) orange juice

125ml (4fl oz) light soy sauce

3 tablespoons honey

2 tablespoons rice vinegar

2 garlic cloves, crushed

2cm (¾ inch) piece of fresh root ginger, peeled and finely grated

2 teaspoons cornflour

PER SERVING
CALORIES 42
FAT 0G
SAT FAT 0G
CARBS 9.3G
SUGARS 7.7G
FIBRE TRACE
PROTEIN 0.7G
SALT 2.2G

This is a popular sweet-and-savoury sauce which is widely available to buy, but also easy to make. Packed with flavour, it's a brilliant quick-fix for meals during the week, or as a flavour boost for a fakeaway. This lower-sugar version uses orange juice for that sweet hit, along with honey for the stickiness, which makes it ideal for glazing and stir-fries. It's also perfect as a marinade, salad dressing or drizzle, or in a wrap.

1   Put all the ingredients, apart from the cornflour, into a small saucepan.

2   In a small bowl or ramekin, stir the cornflour into about 2 tablespoons cold water to form a smooth mixture. Add this to the saucepan.

3   Bring the sauce to the boil, stirring as it heats. Once it's bubbling, reduce the heat to a gentle simmer and cook for 10 minutes, stirring regularly as it thickens to prevent it sticking or catching on the pan.

4   Pour into a storage container. I use an old jam jar if it's going to be stored in the refrigerator, or to store it in the freezer I use small, airtight plastic containers. You can keep this stored in the refrigerator for up to 1 week, or in the freezer for up to 6 months.

WEEK 1 MEAL PLAN

✓ MONDAY > GNOCCHI~TOPPED
VEGGIE COTTAGE PIE (SEE PAGE 22)

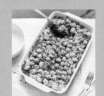

✓ TUESDAY > MEDITERRANEAN~STYLE
FISH WITH GREMOLATA (SEE PAGE 46)

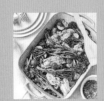

✓ WEDNESDAY > CREAMY BASIL
AND SUNDRIED TOMATO CHICKEN
TAGLIATELLE (SEE PAGE 65)

✓ THURSDAY > SIMPLE RED LENTIL
DAL (SEE PAGE 110)

✓ FRIDAY > BEEF AND BLACK BEAN
BURGERS WITH HOT CORN SALSA
(SEE PAGE 131)

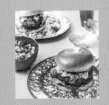

✓ SATURDAY > CHICKEN AND SWEET
POTATO SATAY HOTPOT (SEE 138)

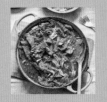

✓ SUNDAY > PORK, APPLE, SAGE
AND LEEK CASSEROLE (SEE PAGE 172)

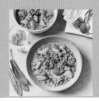

WEEK 1 SHOPPING LIST

FRUIT / VEG

6 onions
2 red onions
4 shallots
2 leeks
garlic
3 carrots
1 celery
1kg (2lb 4oz) sweet potatoes
650g (1lb 7oz) potatoes
2 large courgettes
350g (12oz) cherry tomatoes
4 peppers (2 red, 2 orange or yellow)
1 head of broccoli
1 packet baby spinach leaves
fresh root ginger
1 green chilli
fresh basil
fresh coriander
fresh parsley
2 apples
3 lemons
1 lime

MEAT / FISH

6 chicken breasts
250g (9oz) lean minced beef (less than 5 per cent fat)
500g (1lb 2oz) lean minced pork (less than 5 per cent fat)

FRIDGE / FREEZER

500g (1lb 2oz) fresh gnocchi
Parmesan cheese
60g (2¼oz) Cheddar cheese
reduced-fat cream cheese
4 frozen white fish fillets

STORE CUPBOARD

spray oil
olive oil
salt and pepper
vegetable stock
chicken stock
300g (10½oz) tagliatelle
4 brioche-style burger buns
400g (14oz) can of black beans
400g (14oz) can of chopped tomatoes
200g (7oz) can of sweetcorn
small jar of sundried tomatoes
pickled jalapeños (optional)
dried red lentils
cornflour
tomato purée
mustard powder
cider vinegar
balsamic vinegar
peanut butter, smooth or crunchy
miso paste
dark soy sauce
honey
mustard seeds
cumin seeds
sweet paprika
chilli powder, mild or hot
ground coriander
ground cumin
ground turmeric
dried oregano
dried sage
dried mixed herbs

WEEK 2 MEAL PLAN

✓ MONDAY > OVEN-BAKED LEEK AND PEA RISOTTO (SEE PAGE 21)

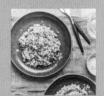

✓ TUESDAY > SWEET POTATO AND BLACK BEAN LAYER (SEE PAGE 40)

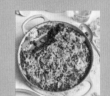

✓ WEDNESDAY > CHINESE 5-SPICE CHICKEN RICE (SEE PAGE 69)

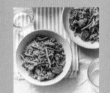

✓ THURSDAY > SPAGHETTI FRITTATA (SEE PAGE 86)

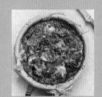

✓ FRIDAY > RANCHERO MAC 'N' CHEESE (SEE PAGE 121)

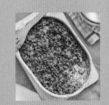

✓ SATURDAY > CREAMY CHICKEN CHANGEZI CURRY (SEE PAGE 141)

✓ SUNDAY > SLOW-COOKER MUSHROOM BOURGUIGNON (SEE PAGE 175)

WEEK 2 SHOPPING LIST

FRUIT / VEG

6 red onions
400g (14oz) shallots
2 leeks
garlic
2 large carrots
2 sweet potatoes
200g (7oz) baby button mushrooms
250g (9oz) chestnut mushrooms
250g (9oz) large flat/portobello mushrooms
200g (7oz) fine green beans
small packet of curly kale
1 red chilli
fresh root ginger
fresh coriander
fresh parsley
2 lemons
2 limes

MEAT / FISH

6–7 skinless chicken breasts

FRIDGE / FREEZER

butter
250ml (9fl oz) semi-skimmed milk
small pot of single cream
150g (5½oz) fat-free Greek yogurt
Parmesan cheese
reduced-fat cream cheese
120g (4¼oz) Cheddar cheese
100g (3½oz) mozzarella cheese
120g (4¼oz) red Leicester cheese
frozen petits pois

STORE CUPBOARD

spray oil
salt and pepper
6 eggs
vegetable stock
chicken stock
cornflour
arborio rice
basmati rice
spaghetti
macaroni
50g cashew nuts
700g (1lb 9 oz) tomato passata
tomato purée
400g (14oz) can of chopped tomatoes
2 x 400g (14oz) cans of black beans
pickled jalapeños
dried porcini mushrooms
200ml (7fl oz) red wine
Shaoxing rice wine
dark soy sauce
nutritional yeast
Marmite, or other yeast extract
chipotle chilli paste
mild chilli powder
Chinese 5-spice
garam masala
garlic granules
ground coriander
ground cumin
ground turmeric
smoked paprika
dried basil
dried oregano
dried parsley
dried rosemary
dried thyme

WEEK 3 MEAL PLAN

✓ MONDAY > INDIAN 5-SPICE SWEET POTATO CURRY (SEE PAGE 24)

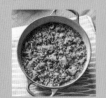

✓ TUESDAY > BLACK BEAN AND CORN LOADED QUESADILLAS (SEE PAGE 36)

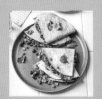

✓ WEDNESDAY > TARRAGON CHICKEN AND MUSHROOM ORZO (SEE PAGE 82)

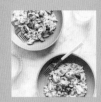

✓ THURSDAY > PARMIGIANA DI MELANZANE (SEE PAGE 105)

✓ FRIDAY > ASAM PEDAS (SEE PAGE 114)

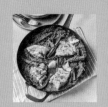

✓ SATURDAY > CHICKEN TAGINE (SEE PAGE 147)

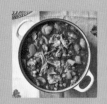

✓ SUNDAY > CHEAT'S CASSOULET (SEE PAGE 168)

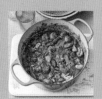

WEEK 3 SHOPPING LIST

FRUIT / VEG

8 onions (including 2 large)
1 red onion
1 carrot
1 celery
3 large aubergines
garlic
2 salad tomatoes
2–3 sweet potatoes
500g (1lb 2oz) fresh or frozen butternut squash
175g (6oz) okra
200g (7oz) chestnut mushrooms
fresh root ginger
1 red chilli
fresh coriander
fresh tarragon
fresh parsley
1 lemon
1 lime

MEAT / FISH

2 skinless chicken breasts
11 skinless chicken thigh fillets
4 reduced-fat pork sausages
1 smoked gammon steak
4 fresh white fish fillets (hake, cod or haddock)

FRIDGE / FREEZER

50g (13/4oz) reduced-fat crème fraîche
120g (41/2 oz) Cheddar cheese
200g (7oz) mozzarella cheese
60g (2.oz) Parmesan or Parmesan-style vegetarian cheese
450g (xxoz) frozen sweetcorn
300g (10 oz) frozen spinach

STORE CUPBOARD

salt and pepper
coarse ground salt
spray oil
olive oil
vegetable oil
vegetable stock
chicken stock
tomato purée
tamarind paste
500ml (18fl oz) tomato passata
red wine vinegar
pickled jalapeños
Dijon mustard
50ml (2fl oz) white wine
dried red lentils
jasmine rice
300g (101/2 oz) orzo
400g (14oz) can of reduced-fat coconut milk
400g (14oz) can of black beans (in water)
2 x 400g (14oz) cans of haricot beans
400g (14oz) can of butter beans
2 x 400g (14oz) cans of chickpeas in water
400g (14oz) can of chopped tomatoes
4 plain tortilla wraps
50g (1.oz) panko breadcrumbs
120g (4.oz) dried apricots
Ras El Hanout
smoked paprika
cumin seeds
brown mustard seeds
fennel seeds
fenugreek seeds
nigella seeds
ground cumin
ground coriander
ground turmeric
dried oregano
dried rosemary
Italian seasoning

WEEK 4 MEAL PLAN

✓ MONDAY > BUTTERNUT SQUASH AND SPINACH LASAGNE (SEE PAGE 18)

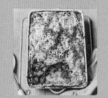

✓ TUESDAY > BACON, LEEK POTATO AND PEA BAKE (SEE PAGE 54)

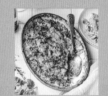

✓ WEDNESDAY > SPAGHETTI FLORENTINE (SEE PAGE 60)

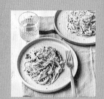

✓ THURSDAY > TUNA AND LEEK PASTA BAKE (SEE PAGE 100)

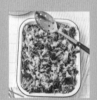

✓ FRIDAY > SWEET AND SOUR PORK (SEE PAGE 126)

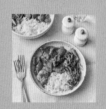

✓ SATURDAY > HARISSA AND COCONUT BRAISED CHICKEN (SEE PAGE 143)

✓ SUNDAY > SLOW-COOKER SCOTTISH STOVIES WITH BRISKET (SEE PAGE 176)

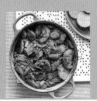

WEEK 4 SHOPPING LIST

FRUIT / VEG

3 large onions
1 red onion
3 spring onions
3–4 carrots
garlic
5–6 large potatoes
900g (2lb) Maris Piper potatoes
1 large butternut squash (around 1kg / 2lb 4oz)
3 large leeks
250g (9oz) cherry tomatoes
2 red, yellow or orange peppers
2 heads of broccoli
150g (5.0z) baby spinach leaves
1 lemon
fresh root ginger
fresh basil
fresh chives
fresh parsley
fresh sage leaves

MEAT / FISH

4 smoked bacon medallions
1 pork tenderloin (about 500g / 1lb 2oz)
4 small skinless chicken breasts (total weight about
    600g / 1lb 5oz)
500g (1lb 2oz) beef brisket

FRIDGE / FREEZER

butter
100g (3.0z) reduced-fat cream cheese
500g (18oz) ricotta cheese
240g (9oz) Cheddar cheese
75g (2 1/2oz) vegetarian Parmesan-style cheese
280ml (10 fl oz) semi-skimmed milk
300g (10.0z) frozen peas
150g (5.0z) frozen spinach

STORE CUPBOARD

coarse ground salt
black pepper
spray oil
olive oil
vegetable stock
chicken stock, including 1 chicken stock pot
beef stock
tomato purée
mustard powder
Worcestershire sauce
brown sauce
cornflour
white wine
light soy sauce
sesame oil
rice vinegar
honey
400g (14oz) can of light coconut milk
2 x 145g (5oz) cans tuna in spring water
432g (15oz) can of pineapple chunks in juice
jar of roasted red peppers
spaghetti
penne pasta
dried lasagne sheets
jasmine rice
harissa paste
dried oregano
dried thyme

INDEX

almonds, toasted 208
apples 172–3
asam pedas (fish curry) 114
asparagus 43, 48, 74–5
aubergine
   & lamb rice, spiced 128–9
   parmigiana di melanzane
     106–7
   teriyaki traybake 48
   tomato & chicken curry
     122–3
   tuna & veg crumble 99

bacon
   barbecue beefaroni 78
   leek, potato & pea bake 54–5
   with stuffed courgettes 53
   see also gammon
beans, black
   & beef burgers 130–1
   & corn quesadillas 36–7
   kale & sweet potato curry
     94–5
   & sweet potato layer 40–1
beans, butter 168
beans, cannellini 92, 220
beans, green
   5-spice chicken rice 69
   king prawn biriyani 117
   miso-maple glazed salmon 43
   spring onions & garlic 210–11
   teriyaki chicken traybake 48
beans, haricot 168
beans, pinto 144–5
beef
   barbecue beefaroni 78
   & black bean burgers 130–1
   Bolognese sauce 180
   brisket, with Scottish stovies
     176–7
   chilli-peanut, with noodles
     132–3
   mac 'n' cheese lasagne 156–7
   Philly cheesesteak-style orzo
     80–1
   pot-roast, with red wine
     gravy 178–9
   & stout hotpot 182–3

biscuits 198, 201, 205, 222
blueberry scones 202–3
Bolognese sauce 131, 180–1
bread, doughballs 158–9
broccoli
   basil, tomato & chicken
     tagliatelle 65
   Mediterranean-style fish 46
   miso-maple glazed salmon
     43
   teriyaki chicken 48
   tuna & leek pasta bake 100–1
Brussels sprouts 150
buckwheat 212
bulgur wheat 28–9, 212
burgers
   beef & black bean 130–1
   pulled chicken 148
   tandoori chicken 70–1
butternut squash 18–19, 147

cabbage 66–7, 105
cake 186–7, 192–3
calories 10
caramelized biscuit spread 188
carrots
   beef & black-bean burgers 131
   beef & stout hotpot 183
   Bolognese sauce 180
   char sui pork 125
   cheat's cassoulet 168
   chilli-peanut beef 132
   & harissa soup 38–9
   mushroom bourgignon 174
   with pot-roast beef 179
   salad 70
   Scottish stovies 176
   sesame shredded salad 215
   sweet potato & chicken soup
     103
   teriyaki chicken 48–9
   Vietnamese-style chicken
   salad 105
casseroles/hotpots 138, 172, 183
cassoulet, cheat's 168–9
cauliflower 30–1, 50–1
celery 168, 179, 180, 183
Cheddar cheese

bacon, leek, potato & pea
   bake 54–5
black bean & corn quesadillas
   36
cauliflower soup 30–1
fried cheese croutons 221
jalapeño popper stuffed
courgettes 53
   mac 'n' cheese lasagne 156–7
   Philly cheesesteak-style orzo
     81
   sweet potato & black bean
     layer 40
   tuna & leek pasta bake 100–1
   tuna & veg crumble 99
chicken
   basil & tomato tagliatelle
     64–5
   cheat's cassoulet 168–9
   Chinese 5-spice rice 68–9
   creamy changezi curry 140–1
   eat-up Sunday curry 162–3
   harissa & coconut 142–3
   honey & mustard muddle
     66–7
   Indian-spiced traybake 50–1
   juicy pulled chicken 148–9
   Korean-style, chilli 44–5
   lemon & asparagus fusilli
     74–5
   Morroccan-style 164–7
   & mushroom orzo 82–3
   pesto & pea couscous 72–3
   & sweet potato satay hotpot
     138–9
   & sweet potato soup 102–3
   & sweet potato vindaloo
     134–5
   tagine 146–7
   tandoori burgers 70–1
   teriyaki chicken balls 144–5
   teriyaki traybake 48–9
   tomato & aubergine curry
     122–3
   Vietnamese-style salad
     104–5
chickpeas
   chicken tagine 147

eat-up Sunday curry 162
Indian-spiced chicken 50
peperonata sauce 92
sweet potato couscous 164
Chinese-style recipes 69, 125
chipotle chilli paste 121
chocolate cracknell 198–9
chorizo 154–5
coconut milk 24, 39, 143, 162
cottage pie, veggie, gnoc-
chi-topped 22–3
courgettes
jalapeño popper stuffed 52–3
Mediterranean-style fish 46
parmigiana di melanzane
106–7
pesto pasta 96–7
tangy tamarind rice 63
tuna & veg crumble 99
couscous 72–3, 164–7, 208–9
cream cheese
basil, tomato & chicken
tagliatelle 65
herby pasta sauce 89, 91
mac 'n' cheese lasagne 156–7
Philly cheesesteak-style orzo
80–1
ranchero mac 'n' cheese 121
rhubarb & custard cake 186–7
stuffed courgettes 53
tuna & leek pasta bake 100–1
crème fraîche 82
croutons, fried cheese 221
crumble, savoury 99
cucumber 105
curry
5-spice sweet potato 24–5
black bean, kale & sweet
potato 94–5
chicken changezi curry 140–1
chicken & sweet potato
vindaloo 134–5
eat-up Sunday 162–3
fish, sour-spicy Malaysian 114–15
king prawn biriyani 116–17
tamarind prawn 118–19
tomatoey chicken &
aubergine 122–3

dal, simple red lentil 110–11
dips 150, 151, 194, 220
doughballs 158–9

eggs 10, 16–17, 86–7
equipment 9, 10
everything seasoning 159, 224

feta 16–17, 27
filo pastry 14–15
fish
Mediterranean-style, with
gremolata 46–7
miso-maple glazed salmon
42–3
sour-spicy Malaysian curry
114–15
flapjacks 200–1
flatbreads, chicken burgers 70
freezing food 10
Fridays 112–35
frittata 16–17, 86–7

gammon 168–9, 170–1
garlic 10
ginger 10
grating 141
ras el hanout mix 226
slow-cooked ham 171
gingerbread treacle muffins
196–7
gnocchi, on cottage pie 22–3
gochujang paste 44
golden syrup 192–3, 198
gremolata 46
Gruyère cheese 109
gyoza, pork 150–3

halloumi, with salad 28
ham see gammon
harissa 38–9, 143
health and safety 4

Indian-style recipes
chicken & veg traybake 50–1
king prawn biriyani 116–17
tandoori chicken burgers 70–1
see also curry

jalapeño 31, 36, 53, 121, 131, 220

kale 32–3, 86
Korean-style recipes 44–5

lamb & aubergine rice 128–9
lasagne 18–19, 156–7
leek
& pea risotto 20–1
pork, apple & sage casserole
172
potato & pea bake 54–5
sweet potato & chicken soup
103
& tuna pasta bake 100–1
leftovers 10, 28, 54, 65
lentils
Bolognese sauce 131
eat-up Sunday curry 162
& kale soup 32–3
simple dal 110–11
sweet potato curry 24

macaroni 78–9, 120–1, 156–7
Malaysian-style recipes 114, 138
measurements 4
meatballs, teriyaki chicken 144
Mediterranean-style recipes
46–7, 98–9
Mondays 14–33
Moroccan-style recipes 147, 164
mozzarella
balls, with salad 28
mac 'n' cheese lasagne 156
parmigiana di melanzane 106
in spaghetti frittata 86
& sweet potato 'sausage' rolls
14–15
muffins, gingerbread treacle
196–7
mushroom
beef & stout hotpot 183
bourguignon, slow-cooker 174–5
bulgur wheat & rocket salad
28–9
chilli-peanut beef 132
Philly cheesesteak-style orzo
80–1

& sausage ragu 76–7
& tarragon chicken orzo 82–3
tuna & veg crumble 99

noodles
egg 132–3
udon 124–5
nutritional yeast 21

oats/oatmeal 200–1, 222–3
oil 10
okra 114
onions
balsamic 17
French onion orzotto 108–9
sweet potato couscous 164
orzo
chicken & mushroom 82–3
chorizo, chilli & pepper 154–5
French onion orzotto 108–9
Philly cheesesteak-style orzo
80–1
tarragon chicken & mushroom
orzo 82–3
oven temperatures 10

panch phoran 225
parmigiana di melanzane
106–7
pasta
basil, tomato & chicken
tagliatelle 64–5
Bolognese sauce 131, 180–1
chicken, lemon & asparagus
fusilli 74–5
courgette pesto spaghetti
96–7
pulled chicken 148
sauces 88–92
sausage & mushroom ragu
76–7
spaghetti Florentine 60–1
spaghetti frittata 86–7
tuna & leek bake 100–1
see also lasagne; macaroni;
noodles; orzo
peanut butter 132, 138

peas
bacon, leek & potato bake 54–5
chicken & pesto couscous 73
& leek risotto 20–1
miso-maple glazed salmon 43
sugar snap 43, 44
peppers
barbecue beefaroni 78
char sui pork 125
chorizo & chilli orzo 154
harissa & coconut chicken 143
hot corn salsa 131
Indian-spiced chicken
traybake 50
Korean-style chicken 44
Mediterranean-style fish 46
peperonata pasta sauce 91–2
Philly cheesesteak-style orzo 80–1
sweet and sour pork 126
tuna & veg crumble 99
Vietnamese-style chicken
salad 105
pesto 73, 96
pomegranate 26–7
pork
apple, sage & leek casserole
172–3
Bolognese sauce 180
gyoza 150–3
stir-fried char sui 124–5
sweet and sour 126–7
tenderloin, with sweet
potatoes & onions 56–7
see also bacon; gammon
portion sizes 10
potatoes
bacon, leek & pea bake 54–5
boulangère 218–19
eat-up Sunday curry 162
honey-mustard chicken 66
pork, apple, sage & leek
casserole 172
salt & vinegar roast 216–17
Scottish stovies 176
sweet potato & chicken soup
103
waffles 22

prawns 62–3, 116–17, 118–19
prep times 10
profiteroles, cheat's 188–91

quesadillas 36–7, 148
quinoa 26–7, 212–13

radishes, roasted 214
ranchero mac 'n' cheese 120–1
ras el hanout 128, 147, 226
red Leicester cheese 78, 121
reduced-fat ingredients 10
rhubarb & custard cake 186–7
rice
Chinese 5-spice chicken 68–9
cooking 118
harissa & coconut chicken 143
king prawn biriyani 117
lamb & aubergine 128–9
leek & pea risotto 20–1
Malaysian fish curry 114
tamarind prawn curry 118–19
tangy tamarind & prawn 62–3
zakkoku 212–13
Rice Crispies 198–9
ricotta 18, 60–1
risotto, leek & pea 20–1
rocket 28

salads
bulgur wheat, mushroom &
rocket 28–9
pulled chicken 148
quinoa, pomegranate, walnut
& feta 26–7
sesame shredded carrot 215
Vietnamese-style chicken
104–5
salmon, miso-maple glazed 42–3
salsa 131, 148
salt 10
Saturdays 136–59
'sausage rolls', sweet potato &
mozzarella 14–15
sausages
cheat's cassoulet 168–9
& mushroom ragu 76–7

scones, blueberry 202–3
Scottish recipes 176–7, 222–3
shallots 175
shopping lists 229, 231, 233, 235
Shrewsbury biscuits 204–5
slow-cooker recipes
    beef & stout hotpot 183
    ginger beer ham 170–1
    mushroom bourgignon 174–5
    Scottish stovies with brisket
        176–7
soup
    carrot & harissa 38–9
    cauliflower, cheese & jalapeño
        30–1
    lentil & kale 32–3
    sweet potato & chicken 102–3
spices
    Chinese 5-spice 69, 125
    Indian 5-spice 24, 225
    ras el hanout 128, 147, 226
spinach
    balsamic onion & feta frittata
        17
    chicken & mushroom orzo
        82–3
    chorizo, chilli & pepper orzo
        154
    lime & jalapeño dip 220
    quinoa, pomegranate, walnut
        & feta salad 27
    spaghetti Florentine 60–1
    & squash lasagne 18–19
    sweet potato curry 24
spring onions 28, 63, 211
steak, cooking 81
store cupboard ingredients 9
stout, & beef hotpot 183
stovies with brisket 176–7
Sundays 160–83
swede 183
sweet potato
    black bean & kale curry 95
    & black bean layer 40–1
    & chicken soup 102–3
    & chicken vindaloo 134–5
    couscous with chicken 164–7
    curry, Indian 5-spice 24–5

    & mozzarella 'sausage' rolls
        14–15
    with pork tenderloin 57
    & satay chicken hotpot 138–9
sweetcorn 36–7, 73, 131
sweets/desserts 184–205
symbols 4, 10

tagine, chicken 146–7
tamarind 63, 114, 118, 122
teriyaki sauce 48, 144, 227
Thursdays 84–111
tofu 105, 126
tomatoes
    barbecue beefaroni 78
    basil & chicken tagliatelle 65
    black bean, kale & sweet
        potato curry 95
    Bolognese sauce 180
    chicken & aubergine curry
        122–3
    chicken tagine 147
    chorizo, chilli & pepper orzo 154
    eat-up Sunday curry 162
    & garlic pasta sauce 88, 90
    hot corn salsa 131
    Korean-style chicken 44
    lamb & aubergine rice 128
    lentil & kale soup 32
    mac'n'cheese lasagne 156–7
    Mediterranean-style fish 46
    parmigiana di melanzane 106
    peperonata pasta sauce 92
    ranchero mac 'n' cheese 121
    red lentil dal 110
    sausage & mushroom ragu 77
    in spaghetti frittata 86
    squash & spinach lasagne 18
    sweet potato & black bean
        layer 40–1
    tamarind prawn curry 118
    tuna & veg crumble 99
tortillas 36, 148
Tuesday traybakes 34–57
tuna 98–9, 100–1
turkey, tandoori burgers 70

udon noodles 124–5

vegetarian dishes 4, 6, 10
Vietnamese-style recipes 104–5
vinegar
    balsamic 17, 27
    roast potatoes 216–17

watermelon & honey lime dip
    195
Wednesdays 58–83
weekly meal plans 6–7, 228–35
Weetabix 196
wine
    red 77, 175, 179
    white 54, 65, 82
wraps, pulled chicken 36–7

yogurt
    blueberry scones 202
    chicken seasoning base 164
    creamy changezi curry 140–1
    in doughballs 158–9
    gingerbread treacle muffins
        196–7
    golden syrup loaf cake 192
    honey lime dip 194
    lemon & mint sauce 70
    minty 128
    spinach, lime & jalapeño dip
        220

GLOSSARY

UK	US
AUBERGINE	EGGPLANT
BAKING PAPER	PARCHMENT PAPER
BICARBONATE OF SODA	BAKING SODA
BLACK TREACLE	BLACK STRAP MOLASSES
CASTER SUGAR	SUPERFINE SUGAR
CHESTNUT MUSHROOMS	CREMINI MUSHROOMS
CHILLI FLAKES	RED PEPPER FLAKES / DRIED RED PEPPER
CHIPS	FRIES
CLINGFILM	PLASTIC WRAP
CORIANDER (HERB)	CILANTRO
CORNFLOUR	CORN STARCH
COURGETTE	ZUCCHINI
COURGETTI	ZOODLES
GRATE	SHRED
GRILL	BROIL
HOB	STOVE
KING PRAWN	JUMBO SHRIMP
KITCHEN PAPER	PAPER TOWELS
MATURE CHEDDAR	SHARP CHEDDAR
MINCED MEAT	GROUND MEAT
MIXED SPICE	PUMPKIN SPICE
PLAIN FLOUR	ALL-PURPOSE FLOUR
PRAWNS	SHRIMP
RED/GREEN/YELLOW PEPPER	BELL PEPPER
ROCKET	ARUGULA
SELF-RAISING FLOUR	SELF-RISING FLOUR
SEMI-SKIMMED MILK	TWO PER CENT MILK
SILVERSIDE	OUTSIDE OR BOTTOM ROUND
SPRING ONIONS	SCALLIONS
STOCK POT	JELLIED STOCK CUBE
TEA TOWEL	DISH TOWEL
TENDERSTEM BROCCOLI	BROCCOLINI
TINS (CAKE, LOAF, MUFFIN AND ROASTING)	PANS
TOMATO PURÉE	TOMATO PASTE
TOPSIDE	TOP ROUND
WHOLEMEAL	WHOLEWHEAT

Acknowledgements

I am so thankful to everyone who follows and supports The Slimming Foodie, whether that's by visiting the blog, interacting on social media, buying the cookbooks, sharing snaps of home-cooked meals, or writing lovely reviews. This wonderful, positive and active community has driven the brand forward. Thank you, I thoroughly appreciate your support.

A huge team works behind the scenes to bring these cookbooks to life. My agent, Heather Holden-Brown and the rest of the brilliant HHB team, Elly and Rob, thanks for all of your hard work. Thank you to Lucy Bannell for combing through the manuscript and ensuring it's all making sense. I'm really grateful to everyone at Octopus for being so lovely to work with, taking the time to listen to me and providing such a warm and supportive environment… I really feel like part of the family now! Special thanks to Natalie Bradley, Anna Bond, Stephanie Jackson, Caroline Brown, Yasia Williams, Sybella Stephens, Lucy Carter, Nic Jones, Karen Baker, Hazel O'Brien and Marianne Laidlaw. And, of course, to everyone else at Octopus who plays a part in the process, as well as Pete Dawson at Grade Design.

I am so happy that the original shoot team has been able to work on this book, they really are the dream team! Chris Terry, Tamsin Weston and Henrietta Clancy, such a talented and fun group of people to work with – thank you so much for being part of this again. Thanks also to the incredibly hard-working Sophie Denmead and Louise Richardson for their valued input on the shoot.

On a personal note, thank you to my husband Darren and my daughters Miette and Marlie for being such a fantastic home team. Thank you too to Sarah and Maria for helping me manage my Facebook group, I am very grateful for everything you do.

ABOUT THE AUTHOR

Pip Payne is behind the award-winning blog, The Slimming Foodie. Her previous cookbooks, *The Slimming Foodie*, *The Slimming Foodie in One* and *The Slimming Foodie in Minutes* have all been *Sunday Times* bestsellers. Pip's passion is creating healthy, varied recipes for the home cook, which are accessible for a kitchen novice, but tasty enough for everyone to enjoy whether or not they are new to cooking from scratch. Pip lives on the edge of Dartmoor, in Devon, with her husband, two daughters and dog.

www.theslimmingfoodie.com

📷 @the_slimming_foodie

f /slimmingfoodie

ALSO AVAILABLE

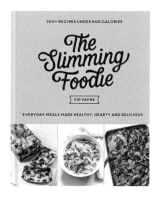 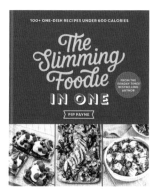 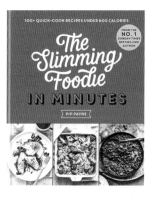